Donna Piazza, PhD
Editor

When Love Is Not Enough: The Management of Covert Dynamics in Organizations that Treat Children and Adolescents

Pre-publication
REVIEWS,
COMMENTARIES,
EVALUATIONS . . .

" . . . Makes an important contribution to the literature addressing organizations that care for and help children and adolescents . . . . Offers a framework that can help researchers and practitioners better appreciate the impact of the unconscious dynamics that are inevitably stirred within these institutions.

The authors also illustrate the ways in which at times seemingly unconnected bits of organizational life can in fact be linked in vitally important ways.

By looking at the unconscious dynamics evoked in these institutions from the 'Organization-as-a-Whole' perspective, this volume makes a valuable contribution to the fields of practice and scholarship."

James Krantz, PhD
Adjunct Associate Professor
The Wharton School

When Love Is Not Enough:
The Management
of Covert Dynamics
in Organizations that Treat
Children and Adolescents

When Love Is Not Enough: The Management of Covert Dynamics in Organizations that Treat Children and Adolescents

Donna Piazza, PhD
Editor

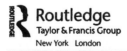

Routledge
Taylor & Francis Group
New York   London

Routledge is an imprint of the
Taylor & Francis Group, an informa business

Reprinted 2009 by Routledge

Paperback edition published in 1997.

Cover design by Marylouise E. Doyle.

Library of Congress Cataloging-in-Publication Data

When love is not enough : the management of covert dynamics in organizations that treat children and adolescents / Donna Piazza, editor.
    p. cm.
    "Has also been published as Residential treatment for children & youth, volume 13, number 1, 1995"—T.p. verso.
    Includes bibliographical references.
    ISBN 0-7890-0223-X (alk. paper)
    1. Child psychotherapy—Residential treatment. 2. Adolescent psychotherapy—Residential treatment. 3. Social groups. 4. Organizational behavior. 5. Student adjustment. I. Piazza, Donna M. 1949- .
RJ504.5.W46 1995
618.92'8914—dc20   95-44786
                                                                              CIP

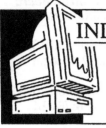

INDEXING & ABSTRACTING

Contributions to this publication are selectively indexed or abstracted in print, electronic, online, or CD-ROM version(s) of the reference tools and information services listed below. This list is current as of the copyright date of this publication. See the end of this section for additional notes.

- *Applied Social Sciences Index & Abstracts (ASSIA) (Online: ASSI via Data-Star) (CD-Rom: ASSIA Plus)*, Bowker-Saur Limited, Maypole House, Maypole Road, East Grinstead, West Sussex RH19 1HH, England

- *Cambridge Scientific Abstracts, Health & Safety Science Abstracts*, Cambridge Information Group, 7200 Wisconsin Avenue #601, Bethesda, MD 20814

- *Child Development Abstracts & Bibliography*, University of Kansas, 2 Bailey Hall, Lawrence, KS 66045

- *CNPIEC Reference Guide: Chinese National Directory of Foreign Periodicals*, P.O. Box 88, Beijing, People's Republic of China

- *Criminal Justice Abstracts*, Willow Tree Press, 15 Washington Street, 4th Floor, Newark, NJ 07102

- *Criminology, Penology and Police Science Abstracts*, Kugler Publications, P.O. Box 11188, 1001 GD Amsterdam, The Netherlands

- *Exceptional Child Education Resources (ECER), (online through DIALOG and hard copy)*, The Council for Exceptional Children, 1920 Association Drive, Reston, VA 22091

- *Index to Periodical Articles Related to Law*, University of Texas, 727 East 26th Street, Austin, TX 78705

- *International Bulletin of Bibliography on Education*, Proyecto B.I.B.E./Apartado 52, San Lorenzo del Escorial, Madrid, Spain

(continued)

- *INTERNET ACCESS (& additional networks) Bulletin Board for Libraries ("BUBL"), coverage of information resources on INTERNET, JANET, and other networks.*
  - JANET X.29: UK.AC.BATH.BUBL or 00006012101300
  - TELNET: BUBL.BATH.AC.UK or 138.38.32.45 login 'bubl'
  - Gopher: BUBL.BATH.AC.UK (138.32.32.45). Port 7070
  - World Wide Web: http: // www.bubl.bath.ac.uk./BUBL/ home.html
  - NISSWAIS: telnetniss.ac.uk (for the NISS gateway)

  The Andersonian Library, Curran Building, 101 St. James Road, Glasgow G4 ONS, Scotland

- *Inventory of Marriage and Family Literature (online and CD/ROM)*, Peters Technology Transfer, 306 East Baltimore Pk., 2nd Floor, Media, PA 19063

- *Mental Health Abstracts (online through DIALOG)*, IFI/Plenum Data Company, 3202 Kirkwood Highway, Wilmington, DE 19808

- *Psychological Abstracts (PsycINFO)*, American Psychological Association, P.O. Box 91600, Washington, DC 20090-1600

- *Sage Family Studies Abstracts (SFSA)*, Sage Publications, Inc., 2455 Teller Road, Newbury Park, CA 91320

- *Social Planning/Policy & Development Abstracts (SOPODA)*, Sociological Abstracts, Inc., P.O. Box 22206, San Diego, CA 92192-0206

- *Social Work Abstracts*, National Association of Social Workers, 750 First Street NW, 8th Floor, Washington, DC 20002

- *Sociological Abstracts (SA)*, Sociological Abstracts, Inc., P.O. Box 22206, San Diego, CA 92192-0206

- *Sociology of Education Abstracts*, Carfax Publishing Company, P.O. Box 25, Abingdon, Oxfordshire OX14 3UE, United Kingdom

- *Special Educational Needs Abstracts*, Carfax Information Systems, P.O. Box 25, Abingdon, Oxfordshire OX14 3UE, United Kingdom

- *Violence and Abuse Abstracts: A Review of Current Literature on Interpersonal Violence (VAA)*, Sage Publications, Inc., 2455 Teller Road, Newbury Park, CA 91320

(continued)

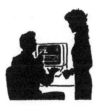

When Love Is Not Enough: The Management of Covert Dynamics in Organizations that Treat Children and Adolescents

CONTENTS

Introduction   **1**
Donna Piazza, PhD

**The Residential Setting in Psychotherapeutic Work
with Adolescents**   **5**
Anton Obholzer

Introduction   5
On Residential Therapeutic Settings   5
The Adolescent Process   6
Containment   7
"Basic Assumption" and "Work" Group Functioning   8
Group and Institutional Processes at Work   8
The Conditions for Institutional Containment   9
Conclusion   11

**Angry Children, Frightened Staff: Implications
for Training and Staff Development**   **13**
Earl T. Braxton, PhD

Selecting and Hiring New Staff   15
Trust versus Control: The Pitfalls in the Agency Setting   17
The Child's Quest for Power   18
Anger and Armoring   19
Angry Children, Frightened Staff   20
The Problem of Fear   21
Holding Environments–For Staff and Clients   23
Strengthening the Therapeutic System   26
Summary   27

Applications of the Tavistock Group Relations Model in Community Mental Health and Protective Service Systems　　29
Ernest Frugé, PhD
Christine Adams, PhD

Part I. Introduction: Core Concepts of the Tavistock Model　30
Part II. Application Case Study 1: Community Mental Health
　　Day-Treatment Program for Children and Adolescents　32
Part III. Between a Rock and a Heartache: An Application
　　of Tavistock Theory and Method in the Context
　　of a Child Protective Service System　41

Revitalizing Human Service Organizations: An Action Research Perspective　　55
Ellen Schall, JD
James Krantz, PhD

Introduction　55
The Method of Inquiry　56
The Underlying Dynamics
　　of Human Service Organizations　57
The Setting　60
The Change Effort　62
Development of a Strategic Theme　63
The Dynamics for Hope and Grandiosity　64
Issues of Leadership　66
Implications for Managers　69
Conclusion　72

The School Romance: Approaches to Subjective Experience of School Life　　75
Daniel B. Frank, PhD
Dennis L. McCaughan, PhD

Desperately Seeking School and the Contradictions
　　of School Life　76
The School Romance: A Paradigm for Understanding
　　the Subjective Experience of the School　78
Transference to the School　81

Idealizing the School: The School as a Stage
    for Developmental Dramas   83
Disillusionment, Loss and Ambivalence   88
Romance and Ritual in the Senior Year   93
The Emotional Structure of the School:
    Towards a Reparative Process   101

ABOUT THE EDITOR

Donna Piazza, PhD, is Assistant Professor in Psychology at Harvard Medical School. She also serves as Associate Attending Psychologist and Research Associate in the Psychosocial Program at McLean Hospital in Belmont, Massachusetts, and as principal investigator, Project on the Development of Personality Disorders at McLean Hospital and the Massachusetts Mental Health Center in Boston. Some of her major research interests include psychological evaluation of personality disorders, psychoanalytic models of female identity development, neural representation of higher cortical functions, and psychoanalytic/developmental models of charismatic leadership. Dr. Piazza is the author of a number of original reports and has given more than two dozen presentations across the country and abroad. She is a member of the American Psychological Association, an affiliate member of the American Psychoanalytic Association and is Vice President and a member of the executive committee of the A. K. Rice Institute.

Introduction

The days of a one person psychology are over. The old-fashioned focus on the individual separate from his interpersonal surround is no longer a tenable focus. Data from infant research, as well as greater cultural awareness and current research in other social sciences, all suggest that the interpersonal and sociocultural contexts of the individual contribute an enormous amount to how the individual is fostered or blocked in terms of what he may accomplish. We live in the embedded contexts of all the groups to which we belong–our families, our places of work, in churches, in leisure and cultural groups, and in our local, national, and international communities.

Children also live primarily in groups–in their families, at school, and in various other community settings. In fact, it is rarely a child's choice to enter psychiatric treatment. He is usually referred by family members, school officials, or some representative of the community, such as the police or the court system. For whatever reasons, the child in treatment has been viewed as not fitting into his milieu–that is, there is an ill fit between the child and one or more of the groups to which he belongs.

Psychiatric treatment usually introduces the child into yet another group–the treatment setting–the hospital, the residential school, the outpatient clinic, or into a new group of two with a private clinician. The persons offering treatment, in addition to relating to the child or adolescent, will also need to relate back to the family, the school, and possibly other groups to which the child belongs. This new treatment group intends to be "therapeutic." Whether or not a treatment setting accomplishes its therapeutic aims depends on a multitude of factors. The competence of the staff, the safety, nurturing and protective elements of the emotional, physical and political setting, and *all* the overt and covert organizational dynamics affect the morale of the group and its ability to work effectively.

[Haworth co-indexing entry note]: "Introduction." Piazza, Donna. Co-published simultaneously in *Residential Treatment for Children & Youth* (The Haworth Press, Inc.) Vol. 13, No. 1, 1995, pp. 1-3; and: *When Love Is Not Enough: The Management of Covert Dynamics in Organizations that Treat Children and Adolescents* (ed: Donna Piazza) The Haworth Press, Inc., 1995, pp. 1-3. Single or multiple copies of this article are available from The Haworth Document Delivery Service [1-800-342-9678, 9:00 a.m. - 5:00 p.m. (EST)].

To ignore organizational dynamics is to court disaster. As in dysfunctional families, organizations can undermine the emotional and cognitive functioning of its staff or the identified patients, and can set serious limits (usually inadvertently) on the growth of the members of the organization, staff and patients alike. Ongoing self scrutiny of the organization concerning its irrational and rational processes is crucial to the health and vitality of the group that purports to offer treatment to others.

These few comments are based on the "Group Relations" model of group and organizational processes that was first developed in the 1940s at the Tavistock Clinic in London. This model was originally based on the pioneering work of Wilfred Bion with small study groups in which he studied such topics as authority and leadership processes in groups, the different roles individuals may take up in groups, as well as the rehabilitation and milieu treatment of psychiatric patients. His thinking was significantly affected by the work of Melanie Klein. His work underlined that the individual's functioning may not be considered separately from the group in which it occurs. The individual may contribute to a group, but the Group-as-a-Whole is a collective entity, in which the work of individuals reflects, in many important ways, the strengths and weaknesses of the group in which the work is attempted.

A. Kenneth Rice is one of the main people credited with bringing the Tavistock model of Group Relations thinking to the United States. He directed the first Group Relations Conference in this country at Mount Holyoke College in 1965. That conference was jointly sponsored by the Washington School of Psychiatry and the Yale University Department of Psychiatry. This and succeeding experiential Group Relations Conferences have focused on authority relations in groups, the development of leadership skills, and on those factors in group life which facilitate or obstruct the ability of groups to design and complete work tasks that are congruent with their stated missions. These conferences are designed for professionals in leadership or training positions in a wide variety of career paths–in business and government, in the church, in the military, and in the educational and mental health fields. The Group Relations Conferences in this country are conducted under the auspices of the A. K. Rice Institute, P.O. Box 1776, Jupiter, FL 33468, and its nine Centers around the country.

The papers in this collection are all informed by the Group Relations model, and are dedicated to the improved psychological treatment of children and adolescents in this postmodern society in which life in our interdependent communities is becoming increasingly important for the survival and health of us all.

SUGGESTED READINGS

Bion, W. R. Experiences in Groups. New York: Basic Books, 1961.

Bion, W. R. Attention and Interpretation: A Scientific Approach to Insight in Psychoanalysis and Groups. New York: Basic Books, 1970.

Kets de Vries, M.F.R. Organizations on the Couch: Clinical Perspectives on Organizational Behavior and Change. San Francisco and Oxford: Jossey-Bass Publishers, 1991.

Klein, E.B. and Gould, L.J. Boundary Issues and Organizational Dynamics. *Social Psychiatry*, 1973, 8(4), 204-211.

Main, T.F. The Ailment. *British Journal of Medical Psychology*, 1957, 30, 129-145.

Rioch, M.J. "All we like sheep—" (Isaiah 53:6): Followers and Leaders. *Psychiatry*, 1971, 34, 258-273.

Shapiro, E.R. and Cart, A. W. Lost in Familiar Places. New Haven and London: Yale University Press, 1991.

Winnicott, D.W. Transitional Objects and Transitional Phenomena. In Through Pediatrics to Psychoanalysis. New York: Basic Books, 1951.

Donna Piazza, PhD
Department of Psychiatry
Harvard Medical School

The Residential Setting
in Psychotherapeutic Work
with Adolescents

Anton Obholzer

INTRODUCTION

Most psychotherapeutic work with adolescents takes place in day settings, be they educational, social service or health service funded and staffed. A significant proportion of psychotherapeutically influenced work with adolescents, however, takes place in residential settings, either because that is where the adolescent is naturally 'resident' on account of 'family difficulties', or because he or she can no longer be contained in the community, and therefore requires admission to a residential setting. There are particular and serious risks associated with work in residential settings, which are geared to work with disturbed adolescents. Whilst this state of affairs is well known to those who work in in-patient adolescent settings, there is surprisingly little written about it, mostly because it is almost impossible to disguise institutions for the purposes of writing papers on institutional processes. The risks are to the adolescents themselves, to the staff, and to the very bricks, mortar and fabric of the institution. This paper will address these issues from a psychoanalytic and organisational consultancy perspective.

ON RESIDENTIAL THERAPEUTIC SETTINGS

Adolescents are admitted to Residential Therapeutic Settings for two main reasons—because they can no longer be contained in the community,

[Haworth co-indexing entry note]: "The Residential Setting in Psychotherapeutic Work with Adolescents." Obholzer, Anton. Co-published simultaneously in *Residential Treatment for Children & Youth* (The Haworth Press, Inc.) Vol. 13, No. 1, 1995, pp. 5-12; and: *When Love Is Not Enough: The Management of Covert Dynamics in Organizations that Treat Children and Adolescents* (ed: Donna Piazza) The Haworth Press, Inc., 1995, pp. 5-12. Single or multiple copies of this article are available from The Haworth Document Delivery Service [1-800-342-9678, 9:00 a.m. - 5:00 p.m. (EST)].

or because the therapeutic benefits of a residential setting are regarded as a necessary adjuvant to therapy. Usually, admission is a combination of both these factors.

Being away from home, or from their usual haunts, is seen as a way of breaking psychopathological bonds, if not permanently, then hopefully for the duration of the admission. Of course, this needs to be balanced against the disruption caused by the breaking of these bonds and the anxiety arising from the ensuing transition.

At the same time, it is hoped that group and institutional processes will work in the service of rehabilitation, rather than in strengthening or fuelling the psychopathological process. My senior colleague, Psychiatrist, Psychoanalyst, former Chairman of the Adolescent Department at the Tavistock Clinic, Dr. Hyatt Williams, illustrates this process with the following simile: Not very long ago, veterinary doctors would administer their medication in powder form by placing the powder on the horse's tongue and then blowing it down the horse's gullet. Occasionally, however, the horse blew first, with imaginable results for the doctor. And so, in work with adolescents in residential settings, it is important not only to decide on the treatment, but to see that it goes the right way and does not back-fire in the way described above, for then the residential setting, instead of functioning in a 'containing' way, would function in the service of fanning up the acting-out process.

THE ADOLESCENT PROCESS

So what are the psychic processes that adolescents are engaged in, and how do they manifest themselves? Based on the introjected experiences of earlier life, the adolescent's task is to begin to lay down the foundations of adult life, particularly in the area of personal, sexual and work identity. This "developmental work" will not only draw on the strengths acquired in childhood, but will at the same time again reveal the weaknesses and flaws of earlier development. Viewed positively, it will also present them for possible review and reworking.

An integral part of finding one's identity as an adolescent is the process of differentiating oneself from what Melanie Klein calls one's "Inner Objects" (generally the parents, as identified with, and laid down in one's inner world). The process of finding oneself starts with a differentiation based on a splitting off from the object. Thus, early adolescent identity is based on *not* being like the parents. This is not the same as having a positive identity; at this transitional phase of adolescent identity, the peer-group and the gang are very important as props–only later does the adolescent develop a fairly secure identity in his own right, and move on to adulthood.

Both the processes of finding one's identity by a rejection of the parental object(s) and of having a peer-group-gang to support one, obviously have important consequences for institutions working with adolescents, for the processes are then re-enacted in the transference with staff and, through the group process, with fellow patients.

Because of the "psychological heat" generated by these processes in the confines of the institution, it is essential that the staff have adequate training, ongoing support, preferably with outside consultancy, and work within a clear-cut management structure with clearly set goals and ideals. In short, what is required is a structure that gives the best possible 'containment' for the adolescent process, as described above.

CONTAINMENT

I use the term 'containment' as used by Wilfred Bion, the psychoanalyst who not only contributed substantially to our understanding of mental processes, but who was also extremely creative in his contributions to understanding group and institutional processes. Bion originally wrote about Container and Contained (and thus the process of Containment) in relation to the mother-child dyad. His thinking was that the child, by a process of projective identification, communicated to the mother its distress. The mother, in turn, took this in, psychically speaking, metabolised it, and then responded to the child in such a way as to give the child the experience of being understood and helped to a degree. Bion called this process 'containment'–clearly a process that was repeated a great many times over, and that eventually led to the development of an inner world in which, by a process of introjective identification, this capacity was laid down. Containment was thus a quality that one developed within oneself in relation to life's pressures.

What Bion described in individual terms, others in England, notably Hyatt-Williams from an adolescent psychopathology point of view, and Menzies-Lyth from an institutional point of view, described as regards the 'containing function of the adolescent setting'. Applied to institutions, this therefore means that the institution as a whole, as an entity, is required to perform the same 'containing' function for the total adolescent psychopathology of its inmates. This is thus the equivalent process to individual containment, but at an institutional level.

At this point, it is perhaps also worthwhile to consider what happens if the containment function does not work. Thus, in the mother-child dyad, if the mother is non- or inappropriately responsive, the child would be left with the feeling that it was not understood, could not be helped; that it was on its own and could rely on no one. Worse still, the situation might arise where, in addition, mother's personal distress would be released by, and added to, the baby's distress, starting a vicious spiral, the sort of process that often leads to baby battering, or to increasing disorganisation and distress in the child.

In its institutional context, this would mean that, not only would the process of adolescent psychopathology not be contained, but might be added to by the adolescent group process and staff psychopathology, leading to acting out, sometimes of a sexual nature, sometimes of a self-destructive nature, and sometimes to the actual destruction of the premises through vandalism and arson.

"BASIC ASSUMPTION" AND "WORK" GROUP FUNCTIONING

In addition to his seminal ideas on containment, Bion also wrote about a spectrum of unconscious group processes. At one end were what he described as basic assumption groups, at the other, work group functioning.

In the basic assumption mode, the group/institution is in the grip of primitive processes of a psychotic nature, processes that are directly contrary to the rehabilitational process that is hoped for in a therapeutic institution. The behaviour of the group at first glance, though, might very well appear to be acceptable; it is only when compared to the concept of primary task, namely, what they should be doing professionally speaking, that the situation becomes clearer. Bion described basic assumptions made of functioning, fight/flight, dependency and pairing. These describe the behaviour found in these basic assumption variants. A group in work mode, by contrast, is in the service of rehabilitation and is on task. As mentioned, this is assessed against the benchmark of the primary task of the organisation.

GROUP AND INSTITUTIONAL PROCESSES AT WORK

Bion viewed the group as a whole–a change from viewing a group as a collection of individuals. From this point of view, an individual is therefore seen, and must be treated as, an aspect of group functioning. Equally, his or her functioning is therefore perceived as, and must be treated as, an aspect of group and *not* of individual functioning. Thus, the adolescent who is caught smoking marijuana in the adolescent unit must be managed as representing drug-taking 'on behalf of the entire group', so to speak. We are thus concerned with a complex network of projective processes at work in the institution. Viewed this way, it is the most "vulnerable-to-drug-taking adolescent" who is unconsciously 'selected' by the group to partake in drug taking 'on behalf of' all the other inmates, as it were. Some of these others might own up to their contribution, others less in touch, or less vulnerable, would deny their part in the collective network of unconscious processes. From a staff managerial process, it would thus be necessary to treat the individual transgression of rules as an aspect of everyone's behaviour, rather than being solely an individual manifestation.

The difference between the two styles of management is of major consequence. Treat it as a group process, and you address the process as such, including the process in the perpetrator. Treat it as an individual manifestation, and everyone else disowns those parts of self projected into the smoker. The latter, in turn, is excluded, or possibly expelled, from the institution, only to be replaced by someone else, and the process continues unabated.

THE CONDITIONS FOR INSTITUTIONAL CONTAINMENT

In order for the institution to be able to carry out its functioning as a unit for the therapeutic rehabilitation of adolescents, certain conditions need to be met, both initially and in an ongoing way.

1. There needs to be clarity of task for staff and patients alike.
2. There needs to be clarity of structure, of authority, of roles, of boundaries.
3. Staff need to have adequate training, particularly in the field of group and institutional processes.
4. There needs to be an awareness of the risks to staff, to the patients and to the institution, arising from the nature of the work in which they are engaged.

Clarity of Task

Without there being clarity of task for the staff about the nature of the work they are doing, it is impossible for them to assess whether or not they are moving in the right direction or succeeding. In work with adolescents, this is particularly important, as confusion is an innate part of the adolescent process. It is therefore to be expected that the confusion will enter the therapeutic staff by a process described by Melanie Klein as projective identification, thus causing the staff to experience the adolescent's confusion. This can be dealt with and contained by well trained staff, always providing that they themselves are clear about their task. If this staff clarity is, however, lacking, the resulting "domino effect" of confusion can lead to confusion of the entire institution and to acting-out that can threaten the entire enterprise.

Clarity of Structure

In order for the staff to be able to carry out their work, it is essential that there is a clear definition of their professional role, and, particularly, definition of the boundary between their and other's role. Equally, the authority and management structure needs to be clearly laid down, and areas of responsibility outlined.

Adolescence is, in part, about finding one's own authority, and learning to relate to authority figures. Adolescent patients in an adolescent unit are likely to bring confusion in this area of functioning to the fore, and can rightly expect that it should be something that staff should be able to deal with. Again, the staff's capacity to metabolise such difficulties is greatly enhanced by a state of mind in which they as professionals have clarity about such matters.

Training

It is well known to all who have contact with adolescents, whether as parents or as professionals, that adolescents have an uncanny capacity to seek any "Achilles Heel," personally and institutionally speaking. This 'exploitation' often takes the form of splitting or attempting to split the parental couple or the coherence of the staff group.

The adolescent's capacity to find such opportunities for splitting is much reduced if the staff group are clear about the above mentioned issues and have a regular, clearly bounded, venue in which to continue work on these issues.

The Achilles Heel, as found by the adolescent, is of course often of a personal nature, rather than an institutional one, and so it is, in my view, essential that certainly the therapeutic staff should have personal therapy or analysis in order, not only to chart their own personal vulnerabilities, but also to get some understanding about the conditions and circumstances in which they are likely to make their appearance.

Thus, informed staff are likely to be less vulnerable to adolescent attack than they might otherwise be, and in addition, have a better chance of "recovery." After all, the successful finding of a vulnerable area in a member of staff, or in the institution, is much less damaging to both staff and patient if they can both be witness to a process of healthy recovery.

What hopefully is therefore introjected by the adolescent is not that adults are supermen or invulnerable, but that they are aware of their vulnerabilities, can learn to live with them, and have the capacity to make a recovery.

In addition to personal therapy, I also believe it to be useful for members of staff to have personal experience of, and training in, the area of group and institutional processes. As with individual dynamics, so with the group–it helps the individual to get some understanding of their personal valency (Bion) as regards group processes, and thus an understanding of which group processes they are vulnerable to, and which less so.

Matters of personal authority, where it originates, how one might manage and maintain it, particularly in the face of hostility and pressure, are also important issues for staff to learn about. They, in turn, can then act as role-models for the adolescents, who are themselves negotiating similar issues of identity, authority, etc.

Risks

Hyatt-Williams, in a paper given in the early 1970s entitled "The risks to those who work with disturbed adolescents," gave a graphic description of the risk to workers. In part, this was outlined above; he particularly spoke to the risk of unresolved and "walled off" aspects of the worker, that perhaps lay dormant in everyday life under relatively little pressure, being detonated by the combined force exerted by individual patients and the adolescent process as such.

Institutions too develop ways of functioning that are sometimes more influenced by the need of staff to protect themselves against the pressures arising from the work, than they are by work-orientated considerations.

As all members of staff are likely to be caught up in this process of institutional functioning, it is often very helpful to have either intermittent or ongoing consultancy from an outside consultant who, by virtue of his outside position, can often bring a different and helpful perspective to the work of the institution.

CONCLUSION

We have learnt from the work of Elliot Jaques, of Isabel Menzies Lyth, of Eric Miller, and of others, that all institutions to a degree structure themselves in such a way as to defend the staff against the particular anxieties arising from the work.

Different areas of work bring different anxieties, as do different age groups. Adolescent institutions have to deal with adolescence as the raw material. Adolescence in western societies is about finding one's identity for future life; thus personal and social, as well as sexual and work identity needs to be addressed. These are all issues that are still 'live' issues in the workers, whether they are young adults, in midlife, or near retirement. The issues are there in the staff–how they are dealt with varies in accordance to age. Thus acting out, envy and a retreat into the above mentioned elements of life are standard staff reactions to adolescent pressures.

The institution and its management can do a great deal to provide a climate in which staff anxieties can be dealt with and contained. I have mentioned some of the issues which we regard as important. If addressed, these in turn give the staff the capacity to contain the adolescents' anxieties, and thus enable both staff and adolescents to carry out the work of the institution.

Hopefully, by the above process, some progress can be made whereby the cycle of deprivation and despair that so many adolescents feel can be broken, so that it is not passed on to the next generation.

REFERENCES

Bion, W. (1961). Experiences in Groups, New York Basic Books (see 'Selections from Experiences in Groups', in A.D. Colman and W.H. Bexton (Eds). Group Relations Reader 1, A.K. Rice Institute Series (Washington DC), 1975.

———— (1962). 'Learning from experience,' International Journal of Pscyhoanalysis, 43: 306-10.

Erikson, E.H. Childhood & Society, Penguin Books, London 1965.

Jaques, E. Social Systems as a Defence against Persecutory and Depressive Anxiety. In "New Directions in Psychoanalysis." London, Tavistock Publications.

Menzies Lyth, I.E.P. (1979). 'Staff support systems: task and anti-task in adolescent institutions,' in Containing Anxiety in Institutions: Selected Essays, London: Free Association Books, 1988.

Obholzer, A. (1987). 'Institutional dynamics and resistance to change,' Psychoanalytic Psychotherapy, 2.3: 201-5.

Obholzer, A. and Roberts, V. (Eds). In "The Unconscious at Work," Routledge, London, 1994.

Williams, A.H. (1971). The risk of those who work with disturbed adolescents. In: Association for the Psychiatric Study of Adolescents. Proceedings of the 6th annual conference, Guildford, 1971. Edinburgh APSA, pp. 71-77.

Winnicott, D.W. (1971). Playing and Reality, London: Tavistock Publications (reprinted Harmondsworth: Penguin Books (1980).

Angry Children, Frightened Staff: Implications for Training and Staff Development

Earl T. Braxton, PhD

Children don't care how much you know until
they know how much you care.

A major problem for the child care field is finding appropriate staff, then preparing and training them to work effectively with troubled children. The pool of applicants includes many well-meaning adults who claim they "like children," and mistakenly equate this with possessing the necessary technical skills to work in the field. Nothing could be further from the truth. Working with disturbed children, especially in residential treatment settings, is a very demanding and challenging undertaking. Commitment to and caring about children is not enough. In a culture that generally under-values its children, those who wish to help tend to under-estimate what it takes to work with wounded children and adolescents.

Unfortunately, funding policies and supervisors' attitudes perpetuate the practice of hiring, and then requiring, the most from the least prepared workers. The pressure on social agencies to maintain programs with limited resources is a key contributing factor to poor service quality and staff burn-out. Agencies often settle for using inadequately trained staff to work with highly disturbed, volatile and vulnerable children. Particularly in

Earl T. Braxton, PhD, may be written at 211 N. Whitfield Street, Suite 490, Pittsburgh, PA 15206.

[Haworth co-indexing entry note]: "Angry Children, Frightened Staff: Implications for Training and Staff Development." Braxton, Earl T. Co-published simultaneously in *Residential Treatment for Children & Youth* (The Haworth Press, Inc.) Vol. 13, No. 1, 1995, pp. 13-28; and: *When Love Is Not Enough: The Management of Covert Dynamics in Organizations that Treat Children and Adolescents* (ed: Donna Piazza) The Haworth Press, Inc., 1995, pp. 13-28. Single or multiple copies of this article are available from The Haworth Document Delivery Service [1-800-342-9678, 9:00 a.m. - 5:00 p.m. (EST)].

13

residential settings, coverage may take precedence over training. Managers may make compromises about staff skill requirements because they feel that a warm body on the scene can at least provide maintenance care, which keeps symptoms under control. In addition, there are few accountability standards for personal qualities of staff such as compassion, sensitivity to children, mature judgment or the ability to manage volatile situations, while controlling one's own anger and anxiety.

The typical, inexperienced young adult entering residential care work with disturbed children has an undergraduate degree at best. He or she is between 20 and 30 years old, and is often in the phase of adult development that involves searching for a personal identity. Since undergraduate and even graduate level educational institutions do little to encourage serious emotional growth, young adult staff with little or no experience working with troubled children are likely to become casualties themselves. They must be given emotional and technical skill preparation for their role as care giver. The responsibility for helping caregivers to develop emotional maturity and childcare skills falls on the supervisors in private and public agencies. However, the development of staff is often secondary to the management of programs and if there are fiscal short-falls, staff training is one of the first items to be eliminated. It is usually a crisis that calls attention to the problem of inadequately prepared staff. For example, a typical crisis situation in residential care is children losing control and hurting people or damaging property. They may run away, steal, become physically ill or exhibit serious psychological or psychiatric disturbances. These types of crises are emotionally stressful, particularly to inexperienced staff. Other signs of a crisis include high staff turnover, low staff morale, and staff who provide little or no therapeutic work with the children.

Inadequately prepared staff may include people with good academic credentials but who themselves lack social or emotional maturity. This type of staff may be more adept at hiding their shortcomings through the use of clinical language and jargon. They often find ways to avoid dealing directly with "acting-out" behavior, and instead intellectually distance themselves by using seemingly sophisticated clinical diagnoses, professional jargon and theories to analyze the child's weaknesses and problem areas. Too often when children present their feelings to these professionals by the only means they know (i.e., angry outbursts, impulsive behaviors, dissociative episodes, or sullen withdrawal, and depression), the professional reaction is predictable. The children are often labeled, medicated, dismissed (abandoned), punished, restricted, shamed, humiliated and/or infantilized. All of this is done in the name of clinical proficiency. Because professionals have control, they can pin all of the pathology on the child, without looking at their own behavior.

We know that troubled children test the inner fiber and character of those who come to work with them. We also know that the child has come to us because he or she was disturbed and needed help to heal the wounds that were caused by the disturbance. These children need to learn alternative ways to manage their internal chaos and anxiety. Staff members who work with wounded children are not paid in a manner commensurate with the demands of their work, but their mission is to provide a therapeutic environment for the children. The staff members are generally expected to work at a "therapeutic level," which includes meeting the child both individually, and in some form of milieu or group therapy. That means that when the child is in crisis, staff members are expected to find alternative ways to help the children to manage their anger, anxiety and pain. We have the right to expect that the staff will rise above the child's limitations. In order to do this the staff person must have inner resources to call on, not just information from books or other people. Staff must have created and built those inner resources before being expected to manage, teach, discipline, love and act as role models for the children.

Managers in charge of hiring must be able to identify the experiences and resources needed by staff, or they will be short-changing those children or adolescents whose emotional healing processes have been placed in their hands.

SELECTING AND HIRING NEW STAFF

When staff members are being hired to deal with children or adolescents, they need to be screened regarding their own childhood or adolescence. There is a high correlation between doing effective work with adolescents and "working through" the problems of one's own adolescence. For example, adolescence is a period of inner (and often outer) turmoil. Normal adolescence brings upheavals such as conflicts with parents, various forms of rebellion, struggles with authority, confusion, sexual urges, and experimentation, to name just a few. No one gets through adolescence untouched, although some may deny the turmoil of it. Moreover adolescence replays the development conflicts of our earlier years, so understanding these childhood conflicts is equally essential. In fact, most people were deeply affected, or even traumatized, by their adolescent conflicts and experiences, and continue to struggle with the residual pain in adulthood. In order to discover the ways in which a person has dealt with personal wounds and conflicts, it is critical that we explore with all potential staff what adolescence was like for them. People who have not come to terms with their own childhood or adolescence will not be open about the conflicts they experienced (during those periods) and they will inevitably lock out the wounded children and adolescents they encounter. They can do even more damage to the disturbed youth if they view the individual through their own unresolved issues, and abuse the authority of their staff position to mistreat the child/adolescent and, in turn, blame the victim.

It is particularly critical to determine how the potential new staff person will handle anger. That may be the most crucial question to explore with any staff person in this line of work. Anger is a healthy emotion and it serves functionally when people are able to manage it, and have a healthy outlet to express it, and do not become frightened by its intensity. Anger has a counter-part and a counter-balance which is the potential for intimacy or closeness. Disturbed children provoke anger because they lack normal outlets for expressing it, and anger is too often their primary feeling. They also defend against closeness because it brings with it feelings of vulnerability. These children will also develop a perception that it is extremely dangerous to be vulnerable in their world. This question should not go unexplored unless we are of the opinion that all anger in the treatment setting comes from the clients, and all staff are above it. When staff cannot face their own anger, they are more prone to mismanage it with adolescents in their care.

Several other important attributes must also be assessed before hiring staff members. The following questions will provide valuable information to the manager facing specific hiring decisions:

1. How willing is the person to look at his or her own personal limitations, weaknesses, and liabilities, as well as strengths, resources and assets?

2. Can the person acknowledge and/or express feelings such as anger, sadness, caring and affection?

   Does he or she understand when, how and to whom these emotions can appropriately be expressed?

   Sample questions:

   • How was anger expressed in your family of origin, and how do *you* express it?
   • How do you behave when you are sad?
   • How do you show others that you care about them?

3. What problems does this person have with authority?
- Describe your relationship with your parents during your adolescence.
- When you had a disagreement with your parents, how did you exhibit those feelings?

4. What is their capacity for intimacy?
- Which parent were you closest to growing up?

5. How well have they managed differentiation from their family of origin? *[This factor is a good indicator of how well the potential staff person can stay out of the child's or adolescent's space without seeming to abandon them.]*
- Who do you depend upon when there is a crisis or problem in your life? Give an example.
- In what way is the relationship with your parents similar or different now as opposed to when you were growing up?
- Describe an important decision you have made in your life and tell how you reached your decision.

When we do not choose staff carefully, the adults we select are often unequipped to manage the children with whom they are charged. The disturbed child frightens the staff because their own feelings are triggered by the child. When they begin working without the ability to identify what their own feelings are, they cannot readily distinguish between their own issues and those of the children they encounter.

Staff Problems–Internal and External

Let us now look at some of the issues and dynamics of troubled children which are the most difficult for staff.

TRUST VERSUS CONTROL:
THE PITFALLS IN THE AGENCY SETTING

Troubled children see the adult world as both a potentially safe, and a potentially dangerous place, depending on how the adults manage the environment. When the adults around them demonstrate that they cannot manage behavior, children begin to feel that their environment is out of control and therefore not safe. When the environment is no longer safe, children behave in dysfunctional ways aimed at survival. If they cannot trust the staff to take care of them, they begin to take action to care for themselves by whatever means available. For some children and adolescents, this translates into flight: that is, they run away if they can, or they withdraw. Others, who see the environment as hostile, take a stance of fighting anyone and everyone to survive. To protect the vulnerable parts inside themselves, they become aggressive and attack with little provocation. There are those who try to out-maneuver staff; their tactic becomes "I'll tell you what I think you want to hear so I can get what I want from you, and stay in control." These children/adolescents are constantly jockeying for a way to stay one step ahead of staff, and are quite good at manipulating the situation. They are often highly skilled at "splitting" staff, which takes the form of getting others to be in conflict on their behalf. The child will often lie, play one adult against another, or take advantage of staff mistakes or misjudgments to increase their power. Losing control is their greatest fear. When children feel they can not rely on the staff to take care of or protect them, they behave as if they are in an unsafe environment. They become more occupied with survival than with growth.

THE CHILD'S QUEST FOR POWER

Normal children and adolescents feel powerless because of their dependency on adults. Under healthy conditions (which presume a relative degree of healthiness in both the child and the adult), children are given increased amounts of responsibility as they get older, and are asked to demonstrate their maturity in handling responsibility. It is a mutual exchange and a gradual process which continues until the child reaches maturity, or moves away from the parents and exercises his or her own internalized controls.

Troubled children and adolescents, particularly in treatment settings, tend to have more intense feelings of powerlessness due to their unmet dependency needs and the high degree of structure required by the therapeutic environment surrounding them.

They have often been disappointed, abandoned or violated by the adults they depended upon and, therefore, are already angry and slow to trust any other adults. At the same time, their need to feel secure and safe is heightened by the continuing threats of their insecure inner world. They manage this dilemma by testing and pushing adults. They seek to test the limits so they can determine for themselves whether they can trust or depend on these new adults in their lives. However, they start from the premise that the adult is untrustworthy, like all the others in their past, and they set out to prove it. It is up to these "substitute" parents to stand up to the test and go the extra mile. This is not easy to do with a child who keeps punishing you for being there while begging you silently not to leave. It is particularly difficult because the adult cannot use the child's overt behavior as the guide post for doing "the appropriate thing"–the adult must have their own inner model of acceptable behavior. Going the extra mile may require either being emotionally available despite intrusive behavior; or it may mean setting a limit for a child who makes you feel like you could not possibly care about them if you don't give in to their wishes. If you cannot meet their demands, or if you leave prematurely, no matter how justified you may be, they will take the position: "I knew you would do this–you see, you really can't trust adults to be there for you." When one adult fails them, all adults come up for scrutiny all over again. Faced with another disappointment the child may respond with uncontrollable rage, withdrawal, suicidal depression–or some extreme behavior that is aimed at hurting self or others.

ANGER AND ARMORING

Anger is the galvanizing emotion of the wounded child whether it is turned outward in aggression and hostile assaults on the environment, or turned inward in deadly, immobilizing withdrawal, depression, or dissociative episodes which are escape routes from overwhelming pain. It is, therefore, critical that any staff person who comes to work with these children must be prepared to work with anger and/or rage (which is a more extreme expression of anger). Anger is the emotion of distancing and separation. The impulse arises in the solar plexus and pushes for release. In more extreme cases, it can result in explosive violence such as physical assault or attack with a deadly weapon. Anger pushes and drives people away. When coming from the wounded child, it is fueled by past hurts and, therefore, is aimed at punishing or hurting a peer or adult in the present. Anger is expressed by striking out, hitting, kicking, biting, scratching, gouging, butting, spitting, or inflammatory and primitive language. Beneath all forms of anger lie the catalyzing emotions of fear, pain and vulnerability. Since the angry child is really a frightened, vulnerable or hurting child, the anger is aimed at keeping people away from the real causations. Expressing or acknowledging the underlying pain and fear often feels dangerous–like giving up one's armor and defenses.

Reich (1972) describes *armoring* as follows:

> Armoring is the result of repeated restrictions of the natural functioning of the body. That natural functioning involves an opening up

to the natural pleasures of touch, contact, and holding with which babies are born, and which many children manage to maintain. The restrictions children experience can range from the normal neurotic constraints on freedom which stem from learned denial of pleasurable sensations (e.g., "Don't touch your genitals," "That's bad," "Shame on you"), to more pathological restrictions such as parental physical and sexual abuse, rigid, controlling and/or rejecting parents; or sadistic punishment and discipline. These restrictions take the form of muscular contractions in the body which cut off the pleasurable flow of sensations and impulses. Temporary contractions occur whenever a person is threatened or frightened by external stimuli, but continuous exposure to such conditions produces chronic contractions which become a reaction to permanent inner rather than outer dangers. Each restriction of the natural functioning becomes a part of character through contractions which unbalance a person and are a response to anxiety, fear of punishment and rejection. As soon as the natural movement expressing surrender is obstructed by an armor block (contractions), the impulse to surrender is transformed into destructive rage. (p. 374)

Rage is a forceful push of energy occurring when the pain from a muscle block leads to tension, then anger. Blocks also cause children to feel inadequate or like failures, and they turn the affirming "yes" into a resistive "no," or "I won't." Depression results when the energy is withdrawn instead of pushed out. The blocked muscles (armor) also lead to distortions about love. What passes for love is often based on anxiety and hate in the armored person, since the natural flow of emotions is cut off. They are replaced by tension, pain, and a constricting inner experience. Love is then experienced as controlling, holding on, and self-gratifying, rather than expansion, release, and freedom.

Thus, our wounded children have great difficulty opening up to love. That is one reason why they are good at "biting the hand that feeds them." They often do not know how to simply "take the hand" of a truly caring adult because this is a completely new inner experience for them, and they have to learn "how" to allow themselves to feel safe or trust again.

ANGRY CHILDREN, FRIGHTENED STAFF

Inadequately prepared staff will often have their own version of armoring. If they do not know how to differentiate between their fear and anger and that of the child, they are likely to take the child's assault personally.

Once the attack is personalized, the therapeutic boundary–the boundary between the child's issues and the staff's issues–is quickly lost and it is only a short step to projecting intent into the child's behavior. When the staff behaves as if the behavior of the child constitutes all of reality, then counter-transference occurs.

In counter-transference reactions regarding anger, the staff frequently acts as if they have no power and no objective authority from which to deal with the child. Frightened staff are the mirrors of the hidden fear in their angry clients. Many programs are not structured to address this problem. It is so much easier to neglect staff and allow them to distort issues when there is no holding environment that will help them to work out their own pain. In the absence of such structures, many of our front-line treatment people, especially in residential programs, become covertly or overtly abusive. Staff abusiveness, if ignored in the short run, will have long range consequences. Eventually these abuses of power cause enough acting out behavior on the part of children to produce a crisis of some sort. The crisis, if examined carefully, has both the child's and the staff's issues contained in it. It is entirely too easy for staff to unconsciously provoke children to act-out, and then blame and punish them. When staff are frightened and have no place to get help and support, they lose control of themselves first, and the children/adolescents they work with next.

Counter-transference–Transference is when the child treats the staff as if they are the authority figures from their past. Counter-transference is when the staff behave as if they are those past authority figures.

Holding Environment structures–Structures that meet the criteria of safety and security to the extent that individuals will risk revealing their inner experiences and covert agendas.

THE PROBLEM OF FEAR

Right next to the child's anger is the adult staff's fear of the angry child. Frightened staff create an atmosphere that feeds the sense of things being out of control starting with that very same staff. The following are some of the effects of fear on adults who work with troubled children:

a. Fear cripples staff and immobilizes their energy.
   Frightened staff cannot trust themselves to act on behalf of the child so they hold themselves back. Disturbed children often recog-

nize the staff's limitations and exploit them. They are, however, in a double bind. That is, they hate the staff for not being emotionally available for them, but they also seem compelled to exploit the staff's weaknesses in order to get control of an anxiety-producing situation.

b. Fear robs staff members of the use of their "observing egos."

Few people are interested in "understanding" what is going on when they are frightened. When staff cannot step back and ask themselves what is happening, and why, they are usually caught in a survival struggle from which they cannot extract the meaning or the message in the child's behavior. As a result, they lose an important therapeutic boundary, and it becomes even more difficult to help the child make different choices.

c. Fear causes staff to engage in survival and control tactics rather than therapeutic interventions.

Frightened staff members will not risk giving a child enough space to solve a problem, either with their help or alone. They crowd the child because of their own fears that things will get out of control, and create "win/lose" situations which are actually losing situations for both staff and child. When the disturbed child has no room to make choices, or is faced with ultimatums and "no way out" power plays, too often they will choose self-destructive alternatives in which everyone loses.

d. Fear causes a split in feeling and thinking.

Frightened staff either become intellectual and lose contact with the child; or they become emotional, and cannot think about the meaning of what is happening. Both positions put staff at a disadvantage with troubled children, whose experience with adults is largely that of being disconnected from them, or attacked by them and not being able to find a whole person when they most need one.

e. Frightened staff are often irrational, erratic, and uncentered.

Even if frightened staff cover their fear, it will not disappear until they learn how to manage it. Being frightened, anxious, or angry with a child is not a problem if adults acknowledge the reality of their own feelings and needs. The feelings themselves are not the problem; it is what the staff do with their feelings that counts. Staff need help in understanding what it is they are feeling and why. When they do not get that help, the children become victimized by unresolved staff issues.

What is needed are structures that enable staff to retain or regain their objectivity and their separateness from the child. Maintaining a therapeutic stance in a treatment setting with children and adolescents involves recognizing that therapy is not an event, but a process. Therefore, being a therapeutic agent requires an environment with structures that are organized around the specific but different needs of children and staff. These structures offer a framework that allows the therapeutic process to unfold over time with safeguards for both staff and children. Offering therapy means creating conditions for change.

Change, if it is therapeutic change, means growth; and growth involves conflict, pain, pleasure, turmoil, and fear. In an effective treatment program, facilitating the change process eventually leads to separation, individuation, and growth. Our wounded children will only risk opening themselves to these emotions and struggles if the agency provides an adequate "holding environment" for them. This can only be accomplished if there is an adequate holding environment for staff.

HOLDING ENVIRONMENTS–FOR STAFF AND CLIENTS

The adequate holding environment as described in psychoanalytic literature is a metaphor for the security of the infant being held by the mother. The holding environment must meet the criterion of safety, without which the disturbed or anxiety-filled person will not risk rectifying his or her condition (Sandler, 1960; Winnicott, 1965). Safety and security must exist in order for wounded children to risk opening up their wounds to self or others. The agency or organization is responsible for the creation of the requisite conditions. Since management is responsible for overseeing the quality of the staff and their work with the children, management must provide an adequate holding environment for the staff in order for staff to create one for the children.

The adequate holding environment for staff in child/adolescent treatment settings has the following attributes:

a. Staff needs the opportunity to come together and express their experiences of frustration and anger with (1) the children whom they are working with; (2) the administration to whom they are responsible. Staff need to have the space for an emotional catharsis about the way in which their young clients impact them and their feelings about the authority figures with whom they must comply. They need to be free to say and express whatever it is that is bothering them no matter how critical, ugly, violent or destructive it may sound. Only after there is genuine freedom to express such feelings can the staff move to the next phase of a holding environment.

b. Once the feelings are out, staff need to be able to find the meaning of their experience. What are their emotions telling them about the problems they are facing? What understanding can they develop by considering what messages are contained in their behavior and that of the children for whom they provide services? The opportunities have a better chance of succeeding if all or at least some of the sessions have an external consultant assigned to them. It is very difficult for the supervisor of a treatment setting to enable the staff to look at the systemic and authority issues that are impacting them when he or she may be a part of the staff's problem(s).

An adequate holding environment for children has very similar characteristics:

> There need to be regular group meetings that encourage them to talk about the problems they are having both individually and as a group in their therapeutic environment both with staff and other clients. They also need to connect current experiences with past events, thereby gaining insight into their own behavior. This then gives them the tools to take more responsibility for their behavior.

Abandonment and intrusiveness are the antithesis of a good holding environment (Modell, 1976). Either of these behavior patterns will produce fragmented and disintegrated systems. Thus, a goal for agency management in providing a good holding environment for staff is to offer them support and listening, without being intrusive. Staff members need a structure to talk openly with each other about the feelings children create in them without feeling judged for having those feelings. Staff, in turn, will be less likely to ignore or intrude on the children who need some of the same things from them. When children's privacy or personal space is invaded, or when frightened staff cannot maintain a therapeutic perspective, then the children tend to lose their boundaries and express themselves in angry episodes, temper tantrums or limit-testing. Unless adult care-givers can help children take more responsibility for their behavior and hold them more accountable, their behavior will become increasingly more difficult to contain. Children and adolescents will not feel safe or secure enough to move past their anger and to openly reveal their more vulnerable, inner selves. Without an adequate holding environment, they will not risk change.

Holding Environment Problems Identified

The main conditions which interfere with the healthy expression of inner experiences in family life, and likewise, in a therapeutic holding environment, are:

a. the depressive condition and
b. the paranoid condition. (Klein, 1959)

The depressive condition is the fear of total indifference from others. It is set off when people in the environment do not pay any attention to the emotional needs of the individual and do not take the time to validate their attempts to express themselves. The depressive condition represents the fear that if I put out what I really feel inside, no one will be there for me. I will be abandoned and/or it will become only my problem and I won't have the means to help myself.

The paranoid condition is the fear of retaliation. "What will someone do to me if I say what I really feel?" It is set off when people attack or criticize staff or children for having the feelings they have, or daring to express them. When the expression of a feeling is treated like a violation or attack on others, then self-ventilation is avoided as a dangerous activity, e.g., "I'll lose my job"; "The staff will hate me."

These issues are related to both the client peer group and the staff peer group. Both of these conditions arise out of a perceived scarcity of caretaking resources* in the larger group system. When these conditions exist, children and/or staff begin competing for what is perceived as a scarce commodity.

It is difficult to correct problems arising from this dilemma and to maintain a holding environment, unless staff are willing to be confronted about their roles. Parents, or staff (who cannot acknowledge their own problems), tend to develop systems (families, groups, etc.) that are unable to be cohesive or responsive. The adequate holding environment requires staff to be available to the child when needed, but not to be intrusive or abandoning. The symptoms we see in systems where children become unresponsive, closed down, or impotently accommodating, are as much a result of flaws in the holding environment as they are a result of an individual's pathology or developmental issues. Training the staff to manage their own anxieties, to work with their fears, and to develop the requisite intervention skills to genuinely help troubled children requires specific training. Agencies often act "penny wise and pound foolish" by cutting the corners on staff training and development, and paying the price in child and staff turnover. An agency is only as strong as the staff who run it--from the administrative level on down.

---

* Caretaking resources, in this sense, are: Safety, love, acceptance, shelter, kindness, warmth, altruistic caring, tolerance for human faults and failings, and ability to "be with" others in pain.

STRENGTHENING THE THERAPEUTIC SYSTEM

There are several staff and agency development strategies that strengthen the therapeutic quality or responsiveness of any treatment system.

1. Use of clinical consultation at the administrative level can help both management and the larger organization to see the broader systems issues, and to carefully determine whether the structures being used are adequate for the tasks being tackled. These include effective problem solving structures that encourage managers to move beyond the limitation of their individual perceptions, and collaborate to examine and resolve systemic and work-group problems.
2. Creation of a support system must include adequate clinical supervision for staff members who provide direct service to the client population. The staff also need the opportunity to share their individual experiences about working with the children and with other staff. They need a confidential, private place to take their own wounds and pains when they are opened up by contact with the wounded child, or by their sibling rivalry and competitive impulses with each other. The wish to look like one is in control by minimizing conflicts and objectivizing issues interferes with the adequate "holding environment." Therefore, each staff level, from administration to line-staff, needs a place where the emotions generated by the work with troubled children can be safely aired and understood. That understanding can then be utilized for taking responsible action.
3. Development of a training plan should emphasize the strengthening of the psychological/emotional capacity of the staff, and then focus on building its skill level and knowledge. The latter is meaningless without the former. No matter how much they know, staff will remain highly vulnerable to the emotional pulls of troubled children (countertransference) when there is insufficient attention given to maintaining staff's emotional and skill development. Moreover, the training must be an ongoing interconnected process, not a series of hit or miss "events." There must be a "training plan."
4. A training program must be ongoing, comprehensive and competency-based, rather than information-based. Competency takes more time to develop, but deepens the staff's abilities and commitment to the work. It focuses on the "how" of behavior, and the skills necessary to get results. (For example: "What does it look like and feel like to effectively calm down a distraught child?").
5. There needs to be a requirement that every staff member be well grounded in child and adolescent development–taught by skilled

practitioners. There is no substitute for this knowledge. Its absence is the source of some of the most destructive staff behavior. A solid grounding in the research findings concerning therapeutic treatment of disturbed children is also necessary for effective functioning on the part of staff.

6. Management training needs to be provided for supervisors and middle management personnel. Supervisors need to have their clinical skills upgraded and new intervention techniques should be taught to improve the quality of the overall treatment process.

Social agencies often ignore good management and create their own turmoil by not managing the work system well, and thereby causing staff disenchantment and casualties. A supervisor who is technically or emotionally unprepared for the task affects many other people, and can interfere with the creation, development and maintenance of an adequate staff holding environment.

SUMMARY

In summary, it is at the service delivery level where the most direct and frequent contact occurs between children and the staff, who in turn must be able to manage their fears and anxieties and make the child's needs their first priority. First of all, staff must be adept at establishing and maintaining relationships with children or adolescents. That is the basis for providing the environmental conditions that allow the child to feel connected and held. Secondly, staff must be able to provide consistency, limits, and loving confrontation to the child, no matter how ugly the child's behavior may be. Thirdly, staff must know where their own boundaries or limits are, and make the child aware of the pain he or she creates for others (including him or herself) without being punitive. In order to do this staff will need training and a holding environment that raises their psycho/emotional capabilities, their skills and competencies, and their ability to translate the child's negativistic or "acting-out" behavior into an awareness of the real issues.

Agencies also need a strong clinical supervisory process, a supportive administrative system, and an adequate holding environment at the staff level in order to meet the needs of the hurt/angry child. Staff development and agency consultation and training can enable systems to develop these structures and processes. Strategies currently exist to help administrative, supervisory, and treatment team personnel to build the needed holding environment for themselves and their clients. The place to begin is by doing an assessment of the staff to find out what they consider as the strengths and weaknesses of their program. They can also be invited to suggest ways the program can be improved. The client system can be interviewed for their own personal perspective. Once the data is collected it may be used to elicit the cooperation of everyone for developing and implementing a plan.

REFERENCES

Braxton, E. "Managing Anger and Anxiety in the Adopted Child." *Adoption Resources for Mental Health Professionals*. New Jersey-Transaction Publishers, 1986.

Gustafson, J., and Cooper, L. "Collaboration in Small Groups: Theory and Technique for the Study of Small-Group Process." A.K. Rice Institute Series Group Relations Reader 2, 1985.

Klein, M. "Our Adult World and Its Roots in Infancy." *Human Relations*, (1959) 12:291-303.

Modell, A. (1976). The holding environment and the therapeutic action of psychoanalysis. *Journal of the American Psychoanalytic Association*, (1976) 24: 285-307.

Reich, W. *Character Analysis*. New York: Simon & Schuster, 1972.

Sandler, J. "The Background of Safety." *International Journal of Psychoanalysis*, (1960) 41:352-356.

Weiss, J. "The Emergence of New Themes: A Contribution to the Psychoanalytic Theory of Therapy." *International Journal of Psychoanalysis*, (1971) 52: 459-467.

Applications of the Tavistock Group Relations Model in Community Mental Health and Protective Service Systems

Ernest Frugé, PhD
Christine Adams, PhD

SUMMARY. This paper describes the utility of the Tavistock approach to understanding group and organizational behavior in two community service settings. It is the authors' opinion that the core principal of the Tavistock Model is the examination of behavior (including thought and emotion) from a systemic or "group-as-a-whole" perspective. Pragmatically, this means that the behaviors of individuals or groups are interpreted as representing the group or organizational contexts of the individual or group being examined. The Tavistock Model is, in essence, an approach to data analysis and does not presuppose specific methods of intervention. Derivatives of the Tavistock Model have been justifiably criticized when applied as methods of treatment. We have found, however, that the systemic perspective on groups offered by the Tavistock Model suggests possibilities of intervention or, conversely, prudent restraint from action not afforded by other perspectives. The Tavistock approach is exceptionally useful in explaining what interferes with well designed, well intended efforts to help children and adolescents with serious behavioral, emotional and familial problems. *[Article copies available from The Haworth Document Delivery Service: 1-800-342-9678.]*

Ernest Frugé, PhD, is affiliated with the Department of Family Medicine, Baylor College of Medicine. Christine Adams, PhD, is in private practice, Houston, Texas.

[Haworth co-indexing entry note]: "Applications of the Tavistock Group Relations Model in Community Mental Health and Protective Service Systems." Frugé, Ernest, and Christine Adams. Co-published simultaneously in *Residential Treatment for Children & Youth* (The Haworth Press, Inc.) Vol. 13, No. 1, 1995, pp. 29-53; and: *When Love Is Not Enough: The Management of Covert Dynamics in Organizations that Treat Children and Adolescents* (ed: Donna Piazza) The Haworth Press, Inc., 1995, pp. 29-53. Single or multiple copies of this article are available from The Haworth Document Delivery Service [1-800-342-9678, 9:00 a.m. - 5:00 p.m. (EST)].

29

PART I. INTRODUCTION:
CORE CONCEPTS OF THE TAVISTOCK MODEL

Theory

The Tavistock approach to group dynamics originated with practitioner/ theorists such as Bion who first interpreted groups as whole systems in terms of object relations theory. Bion conceptualized the difficulties of joining with others to do work in a group as similar to the developmental challenge an infant faces in negotiating the relationship with the maternal object. For example, from this perspective, the anxiety associated with the threat of losing one's identity in joining a group can lead to splitting, destructive competition for leadership and autonomy or, conversely, mindless merging with charismatic leaders. More recent theoretical formulations focus on socio-political or inter-group processes such as those seen in racial and ethnic struggles and biases.

We think the Tavistock conceptualization of task, authority, role, boundary and representation is particularly helpful in understanding the dynamics of groups in complex clinical settings. From a Tavistock perspective, groups come into being for the purpose of accomplishing something: the group's specific or primary task. The nature of these tasks varies widely but all aspects of a group's structure and function can be characterized according to the relationship they have to the primary task of the group. The Tavistock perspective leads one to ask, "Do the existing structures or functions help or hinder the task?"

Authority is defined as the right to do work. Some rights (and thus authority) are personal or universal, but the critical issue in most organizations is determining how this right–this authority–is delegated within the institution. We ask "From where does this authorization originate and what is its scope?" The key concepts of role, boundary and representation refer to the way groups configure the activities of members or sub-groups. Role generally refers to a range of behaviors or a function that is assigned to an entity. Boundary generally refers to the limit of a role, its scope of authority or responsibility. Most work in organizations involves transactions across boundaries. The way in which roles, both for individuals and groups, are structured and interact around the primary task determines the boundaries of a system. Appropriate boundaries can support productivity while blurred boundaries can lead to confusion of authority, muddled accountability and chaos.

From a Tavistock perspective, all transactions are conducted by people who are representatives of groups in one way or another. When there are problems in role performance or in the transactions between roles, a Tavistock perspective would suggest that the difficulties might reflect the influence of unconscious motivations and conflicts that exist in and between the larger groups represented in the particular encounter. In addition to theories about the impact of groups on individuals, the theory also assumes that individuals have personal characteristics which manifest themselves as propensities or "valencies" for certain types of behavior within a group (i.e., consensus builder, devil's advocate, etc.). These valencies can emerge in a group context which either "pulls" for that behavior or does not regulate its expression through organizational structures.

Even though Tavistock interpretations of an individual's behavior within a group are based on understanding the dynamic group context, individuals are held accountable for their own actions. For example, an acting out adolescent may be pulled into his/her typical role of "rebel against authority" in a therapy group. The systemic nature of the Tavistock model would prompt the therapist to consider not only the individual's personality characteristics, but also what group dynamics interfere with the child learning how to negotiate more appropriately with authority figures and what group dynamics would provoke this child into an ineffective, prototypical pattern of behavior. Although the child is still held accountable for his/her own actions, descriptions and interpretations of the group level dynamics that evoke redundant, maladaptive responses are used to help the child learn to exercise better judgment and self-control. Interpretations are also used to minimize viewing the inappropriate behavior as exclusively a manifestation of the child's "pathology."

Practice

The first step in applying the Tavistock perspective is to ascertain the nature and level of clarity in definition of the primary task of the organization(s) involved in a particular context. This includes the "organization of origin" of the observer. Once the primary tasks are defined, then the behaviors of the participants are examined as to whether they are in line or support the work towards the primary task. Structurally, we ask if the roles and boundaries in an organization are delineated in ways that rationally fit the task of the organization. Functionally, we examine how the behavior of people within the system conforms to the delegation of authority within roles and the consciously delineated purpose of transactions which occur at the boundaries between roles. When difficulties emerge within the conduct of individuals in roles or in the transactions at the boundary between roles, the Tavistock perspective leads us to examine how the discrepancies and perturbations are representative of something about that particular sector of the organization, the nature of the interacting groups or the institution as a whole. Our own responses to the situations, including the interpretations we make of the surrounding conditions, is also thought of as representing something about our own group, the organization it represents and the interaction of groups in context.

The Tavistock model proposes that rational organizational structures attenuate interference from unconscious individual and group dynamics. Rational structure means that the tasks of a group are clearly defined and that each person is assigned a task (role) based on competency to do the work. It is the authors' opinion that irrational, often unconscious, individual and group dynamics interfered with the positive functioning of the two groups used as case illustrations. The first case study demonstrates how individual characteristics or personal valencies can impinge on effective work when organizational structure is eliminated. The second case study addresses how overall functioning improved within an organization after a rational organizational structure evolved.

PART II. APPLICATION CASE STUDY 1: COMMUNITY MENTAL HEALTH DAY-TREATMENT PROGRAM FOR CHILDREN AND ADOLESCENTS

Task and Structure of the Day Hospital Program

The first application took place in the context of a Day Hospital program within a private non-profit child mental health center. We will track the experience of a female psychologist from the time she joined the organization to the point of her resignation. For convenience, we hereafter refer to the psychologist as "PSY" and the parent organization as CMHC. The mission and general structure of the DAY HOSPITAL program was similar to most child and adolescent Day Hospital programs in the United States. The goal of the DAY HOSPITAL program in this institution was to provide a cost-effective intermediate alternative to more expensive and restrictive hospital and residential treatment programs for children and adolescents. Most children came from single parent families. The ethnic and racial mix was fairly representative of the city at large. Most families had modest incomes but a few were indigent or wealthy. Occasionally the children were in the custody of Protective Services with mandated parental involvement, but most families were in treatment voluntarily.

The most common principal diagnoses were Disruptive Behavior Disorders. The next most common diagnosis was Depression. Most of the children admitted to the DAY HOSPITAL program had a history of chronic academic and behavioral problems in school. Approximately 30% of the children had a diagnosis of specific learning disabilities. It is also interesting to note that while reading difficulties are most common in the general population, the learning disabilities of this DAY HOSPITAL population predominately involved math and writing.

When PSY joined the staff as a part time supervising psychologist, the DAY HOSPITAL program had been a successful division of the CMHC institution. In fact, it was one of the few programs which consistently generated income for the entire parent organization. The director of the DAY HOSPITAL program, DR-1, was the original designer of the DAY HOSPITAL program and purposely developed a strong educational component. She had hired EDC who had extensive experience in special education to be the educational coordinator for the program.

While the DAY HOSPITAL program had an unusually strong academic component, it had a less developed psychotherapy component. The educational staff was comprised of experienced educators; the psychotherapy staff was comprised mostly of recent graduates of master's degree programs or trainees from local social work, education or psychology programs. The director had recruited PSY to "upgrade the therapy component of the program." One afternoon a week, the director also had the services of a consulting psychiatrist who was an exceptionally competent child and family therapist.

The DAY HOSPITAL program lines of authority initially were as follows: PSY supervised the staff therapists and any trainees assigned cases in DAY HOSPITAL; the educational coordinator, EDC, monitored the educational component and supervised teachers hired by CMHC (but not the teachers provided by the school district) and the "psych techs." Both PSY and EDC reported to DR-1. The consulting psychiatrist's role was to evaluate, prescribe and monitor medication for patients. The psychiatrist also had the authority to discharge patients to more restrictive settings. He maintained a consulting, non-supervisory role with respect to psychotherapy. Staffings of patients on medication included the psychiatrist and all staff who were involved in that patient's care.

Initial Interpretations and Interventions

Upon entry, PSY found the DAY HOSPITAL program to be well run and successful with only two apparent difficulties. The first was some ambiguity in task definition and the second involved disruptive intrusions from another CMHC program, the RAPID RESPONSE TEAM. The primary task of the Day Hospital program vis á vis the child guidance institution (CMHC) was clear. This was to fill a step in a comprehensive continuity of care system so as to insure the economic viability of the CMHC institution. The primary task of the DAY HOSPITAL program for the benefit of patients, however, was not so clear. The composition of the DAY HOSPITAL staff, being strongly weighted towards education, led to ambiguity as to whether the focus of the program was special education or psychotherapy. The combination of developmental, disruptive behavior and mood disorders displayed by the patients amplified the confusion caused by the ambiguity of task and further interfered with appropriate integration of services for overall care.

In order to clarify that the primary task of the DAY HOSPITAL program was mental health treatment without losing the benefits of the strong educational component, PSY suggested that the definition of the primary task of DAY HOSPITAL be made congruent with the central developmental challenge faced by the children in the program. She conceptualized this task as helping the children gain the requisite knowledge and social skills to be successful, autonomous citizens of the community. The work of school was thus defined as the developmentally essential "work" of the children and a venue for the development of the knowledge base and general skills of self-control and discretion crucial to self-sufficiency.

Success in school tasks and the behaviors requisite for this success came to be primary goals and were integrated with more traditional mental health objectives such as enhanced mood, durable self-esteem and improved relations with family and peers. For example, individual and family therapy treatment plans came to include a focus on helping children develop academic skills and task persistence, helping parents form accurate expectations about the child's academic abilities and constructing family-based incentive systems that interlocked with school performance. When the primary task was clarified, the DAY HOSPITAL organizational structure worked well because it already had clear lines of authority, clear task and role definitions, and appropriate intragroup boundaries around tasks and roles.

At this time, PSY applied the Tavistock perspective mainly to the work with family systems, group therapy sessions and to address the problem of intrusions from the RAPID RESPONSE TEAM. Training in experiential conferences in the Tavistock tradition provides practice at stepping back from intense emotional encounters and asking how these experiences pertain to the task at hand and reflect issues in the whole group or groups represented. It helped PSY to view the DAY HOSPITAL patients not only as "members of the DAY HOSPITAL community," but also as delegates from troubled families where collaborative problem solving and constructive conflict negotiation were absent or minimal and coercion was the norm of interaction. The provocative effects of the patients' repertories on the staff were observed in all the therapy formats as well as school. Therapists, teaching staff and administrators were repeatedly pulled out of role and responded in authoritarian, non-empathic ways that replicated the hostile, coercive styles imported by the patients from their family experience.

The Tavistock approach helped shift the focus from blaming an individual child (or staff for that matter) as the "trouble maker" to examining how patterns of behavior were similar to patterns within the child's family. The basic intervention involved examining how the individual's behavior either represented a concern shared by all (perhaps unconsciously) or, as in the case of intrusions from the RAPID RESPONSE TEAM, how a colleague's disruptive behavior represented the lack of clear organizational structures to support tasks and roles. This examination minimized scapegoating and assisted with problem resolution.

A Brief History of the Organizational Times

Readers interested in a more detailed history of the parent organization from a Tavistock perspective may contact the authors. A brief synopsis is as follows: As a non-profit institution, a large source of funding for the parent CMHC institution came from direct and indirect charitable contributions. When the local economy went through a dramatic decline, revenues to the institution declined proportionately. The CMHC institution saw a concomitant increase in demand for services from patients with low or no incomes. The CMHC Board of Directors became realistically anxious about the financial viability of CMHC. A charismatic child psychiatrist was hired as Director of CMHC to "save" the institution. This leader brought a personal friend on board and together they promoted a new model for CMHC's delivery of services to families in crisis. This program, the RAPID RESPONSE TEAM, was touted as being on the cutting edge of new treatment modalities that would bring the institution through troubled times with a more entrepreneurial approach to the realities of an increasingly competitive health care market.

The Director of CMHC and his associate secured a five year grant from a private foundation to develop and implement the new RAPID RESPONSE TEAM model which resembled Multiple Impact Therapy. The model required the availability of multiple staff at short notice. Some senior CMHC staff questioned the cost-effectiveness of this model. A deep split evolved within the institution with the sides roughly characterized as being aligned with or against the charismatic leader. Many staff left or were terminated. Newly recruited staff adopted the view of the director about the specialness of the new RAPID RESPONSE TEAM.

Within three years, the RAPID RESPONSE TEAM had used all five years of its grant funding and had to be subsidized by the other CMHC programs. However, most of the remaining CMHC staff did not openly question the rationality of the RAPID RESPONSE TEAM and the continuation of its preferred status. The priority given to the RAPID RESPONSE TEAM led to recurrent problems in maintenance of boundaries between services in terms of staffing and resources. Other programs were given less resources even though their economic and treatment records were sound.

Within this context, the CMHC director resigned as a result of an ongoing conflict with the CMHC Board over the financial state of the center. A board member with no mental health experience was hired as a replacement and titled Administrative Director. A psychiatrist was hired as Medical Director to oversee clinical services. Within months the DAY HOSPITAL director, DR-1, resigned, having become weary of fighting for resources for the DAY HOSPITAL program and against the ongoing disruptive intrusions from the RAPID RESPONSE TEAM. The new Medical Director hired a psychiatric nurse, DR-2, as the new DAY HOSPITAL director. DR-2 had worked with the new Medical Director in another organization and had prior experience in non-profit inpatient psychiatric facilities. Her prior management experience was as a head nurse of a psychiatric inpatient unit.

Deconstruction

In the first year of DR-2's directorship of the DAY HOSPITAL program, the structure remained unchanged. During this time period, despite shrinking healthcare dollars at large, the program census was high and behavior problems presented by the patients were relatively minor and manageable. The morale of staff was high. DR-2 was instrumental in clarifying and strengthening the mental health skills of the psych techs which made the entire mental health component stronger.

After her first year as director, DR-2 decided unilaterally to flatten the DAY HOSPITAL hierarchy and have all staff, both educational and therapeutic, report directly to her. Ostensibly this change was made as a move towards a more collegial atmosphere and so that DR-2 would not be isolated from actual service delivery. DR-2 said that she thought that all staff were on an equal level with one another and that she was "just administratively responsible" for the program. She removed the consulting psychiatrist from all team meetings saying he "just made staff anxious." Each therapist individually updated him on all relevant cases. The psychiatrist became functionally isolated from the program as a whole.

DR-2 then began to miss work frequently and was later diagnosed with chronic fatigue syndrome. The program became chaotic and staff were confused about lines of authority, supervision and responsibility. Without a hierarchy of decision-making authority, decisions were delayed or inappropriate, adding to the confusion and frustration. The census dropped dramatically and the behavior of patients became unmanageable. For example, the census dropped from an average of 26 patients to about 10 while the occasions where patients required physical restraint ("holdings") increased from 3 to 54 in a comparable month from the previous year. PSY thought the dysfunction of the program was related to the collapse of structure. PSY repeatedly pointed out the correlation between increased chaos and the lack of staff structure. The DAY HOSPITAL director, DR-2, would verbally agree that more structure was in order but never took action to reinstate it.

As the situation continued to deteriorate without change in sight, PSY wrote a memo to DR-2 simply describing the structure from the previous year with the census and physical restraint figures and compared it with existing structure, census and physical restraint figures. Copies of the memo were also sent to DR-2's immediate supervisor and the administrative director of CMHC. Soon after, DR-2 went on a medical leave of absence. A junior Ph.D. level psychologist (DR-3) with no management experience was appointed acting director of DAY HOSPITAL. He decided not to alter the existing, flattened hierarchy, saying that he did not want to change the structure in case DR-2 returned soon. The problems in patient behavior continued to escalate into more violent outbursts and PSY resigned.

Summary Interpretations

In the absence of appropriate delineation of roles and delegation which authorizes individuals to do work within clearly defined boundaries and accountability, irrational processes usually become more influential. The course of the DAY HOSPITAL program offers a clear example of how these irrational, unconscious processes can impact the delivery of clinical services when organizational structures become confused or determined by anxiety rather than the institutionally authorized task. Clarification of the task of the DAY HOSPITAL program proved to be the simplest diagnosis and appeared to lead to positive integration of the DAY HOSPITAL program. Factors within the larger institution of CMHC, however, set a context which allowed irrational personal and group dynamics to ultimate-ly supersede these gains.

Personal Factors

It is an important point that each time the DAY HOSPITAL director position was open after DR-1 resigned, PSY would have been appointed to it if she had been willing to become a full time employee. Because of her family developmental cycle, full time work was not an option. This in effect placed each of the subsequent directors in a supervisory role over someone with far more experience and seniority in clinical and organiza-tional work. This was also the case with respect to the educational coordi-nator who was far more knowledgeable than anyone in DAY HOSPITAL about the educational needs of learning disabled children and classroom management of special needs children.

The personal challenge of supervising more senior professionals may have been one reason that, in spite of a track record of success with one DAY HOSPITAL structure, neither of the two subsequent DAY HOSPI-TAL directors returned to that structure. Both DR-2 and DR-3 were nov-ices relative to the educational coordinator and PSY. It is likely that their decision to not employ a hierarchy of differentiated roles was more deter-mined by their personal reluctance to delegate their authority to experi-enced clinicians and educators rather than the suitability of the flat struc-ture to the tasks of the DAY HOSPITAL program. The result was inefficiency and frustration. Both directors became overburdened by their span of management responsibilities, both failed to discriminate between directorial and staff responsibilities, and experienced team members were not utilized at their highest level of competency.

One obvious example of the problems caused by the ambivalence around delegation emerged when a new staff member, NSM, was added to the team. PSY was the only professional at that time in the DAY HOSPI-TAL program who had legal authority to sign insurance claim forms. PSY had informed the director that she could sign insurance forms only for those cases where she had direct supervisory control. Despite having been given this information, DR-1 then told the new staff member, NSM, that she (NSM) had complete clinical authority over cases assigned to her. PSY was not notified of this communication. Not surprisingly, NSM was of-fended when PSY attempted to supervise her work. Both DR-2 and NSM were irritated when PSY maintained her refusal to sign insurance forms on any DAY HOSPITAL cases where she was not the designated supervisor of the case.

The lack of a hierarchy of supervision and clinical decision making authority reduced quality of patient care since staff of greater expertise such as PSY, EDC, and the consulting psychiatrist had no delegated authority to direct treatment decisions. With the emphasis on "we are all the same here" new staff would not consult more experienced staff. They would make therapeutic interventions that contradicted other staff or were simply erroneous due to lack of knowledge or experience. Another example occurred when PSY's clinical decision not to admit an actively psychotic child to the DAY HOSPITAL program was overruled by DR-2. The reason given was that DR-2 "felt sorry" for the parents. The child was too severely disturbed for the DAY HOSPITAL program to manage and had to be discharged to the county psychiatric hospital as an emergency.

Another personal characteristic that might have led DR-2 to flatten the educational hierarchy in particular became apparent early on in her tenure. DR-2 was very uncomfortable with the strong educational component of the program. She frequently commented that DAY HOSPITAL was not a school. Eventually it was learned that growing up she had had adversive educational experiences. This might have led to a covert, anti-education sentiment. The flattened hierarchy took away EDC's authority over some aspects of classroom management. EDC could no longer draw a boundary around who was authorized to give recommendations to teachers and psych techs. This situation permitted multiple, inexperienced therapists to give unsupervised, uncoordinated input. Classroom management became confused and the children became increasingly more disruptive. Since females held many of the leadership positions described thus far, a case could be made that the problems were a reflection of the difficulty women sometimes have in supporting and collaborating with other women in authority. However, since the same issues emerged with a male director and the male psychiatrist's competence was also underutilized, issues of competition between women could not have been the only factors. There were also examples of individuals who were able to exercise their personal authority and perform competently in spite of significant irrational dynamics in the group and institution. The educational coordinator, EDC, was confident of her skills, task oriented and clear about the boundaries of her role and expertise. These and other personal characteristics allowed her to stay on task even after the hierarchy was flattened and her delegated authority curtailed.

Institutional Factors

Group dynamics in the larger institution impact the ability of staff to remain in role. An example of institutional countertransference and an interpretation based on that process occurred in a community meeting after the DAY HOSPITAL program was going through its tremendous upheaval. As stated before, the Tavistock perspective also leads to the question, "What is being expressed that is shared by all?" This question permitted the formulation of empathic interpretations that included the experience of both staff and patients. Staff at that time were experiencing lack of support and stability from the parent organization and the DAY HOSPITAL structure itself. An argument arose in one meeting with four adolescents who were seated together complaining about a psych tech's enforcement of a rule. The DAY HOSPITAL director at the time, DR-3, became irritated and, in essence, told them "That's the rule; like it or lump it." PSY made a modest interpretation that no one, patient or staff, likes unfair rules or treatment. The effect was striking. The entire row of four adolescents representing the patient complaints all visibly relaxed and sat back as a unit. The discussion then proceeded to more constructive problem-solving and clarification of rules for all concerned.

The interpretation probably worked at one level because the children's concerns about being mistreated were acknowledged as legitimate and normalized as a universal concern, thus averting a power struggle. We speculate that the interpretation also worked at another level by linking the staff's institutional experience with that of the patients in an empathic way. This in turn fostered reflection and permitted an objective appraisal of the situation and facilitated a return to a task appropriate role. This example highlights how the institutional experience of staff can contribute to countertransference, in this case making it easy for DAY HOSPITAL staff to get into a power struggle with the patients about unfair treatment rather than respond more therapeutically. The dynamics in the subsequent staff meeting are particularly interesting. PSY proceeded to explain the community group dynamics to the staff and give DR-3 unsolicited and unauthorized "supervisory feedback" in front of the entire staff about his "unhelpful" interchanges with the adolescents. Later, DR-3 appropriately confronted PSY for undermining his authority by criticizing his work in front of other staff. It is quite possible that at this point in time PSY was becoming frustrated with the state of the program and was being covertly competitive by "showing off" her expertise in a patronizing manner.

There was lack of coordination between the two female directors of Day Hospital and RAPID RESPONSE TEAM DR-2 and RR-1. This led to confusion and competition about who was responsible for cases where both services were involved. For example, a RAPID RESPONSE TEAM trainee had a case which was admitted to DAY HOSPITAL. The trainee actively resisted supervision from PSY even though PSY was designated as the DAY HOSPITAL supervisor for this case. Interestingly, for several weeks PSY was not informed by anyone that she was supervising the case. Input from the consulting psychiatrist was also resisted by the trainee despite the fact that he was legally responsible for the medication component of care as well as an excellent teacher.

Being familiar with the Tavistock approach often helped PSY pull back from immediate and confusing pulls of various groups in DAY HOSPITAL and reflect on a course of action based on her understanding of task and role. Even though this knowledge enhanced PSY's personal performance and coping with organizational strains, she was not immune to powerful group dynamics and unconscious motivations. There were definitely times when PSY engaged in covert maneuvers for leadership and influence beyond her institutionally authorized role. PSY's knowledge of Tavistock principles helped her realize when she was out of role, overstepping her authority or intruding on others' boundaries and then helped her get back on task. It certainly assisted with making sense of seemingly absurd processes and decisions.

It is noteworthy that serious problems persisted after PSY's resignation. DR-2 was permanently replaced by DR-3 as the DAY HOSPITAL director and he maintained a flat hierarchy of authority. This prompted his immediate supervisor to give him a copy of the memo previously mentioned that PSY had written to DR-2 describing the successful program and its structure and the problematic program and its structure. Eventually, a new hierarchical structure evolved with the creation of an administrative director of DAY HOSPITAL, DR-4, and a psychiatrist appointed as the medical director of DAY HOSPITAL with complete supervisory authority over all clinical decisions. Education was relegated to the role it traditionally plays in inpatient psychiatric facilities and the educational coordinator position was eliminated.

PART III. BETWEEN A ROCK AND A HEARTACHE: AN APPLICATION OF TAVISTOCK THEORY AND METHOD IN THE CONTEXT OF A CHILD PROTECTIVE SERVICE SYSTEM*

The second application of the systemic Tavistock approach takes place in a public sector organization serving abused and neglected children and their families. In addition to highlighting some of the organizational complexity that characterizes institutions operating in the public sector, the case study also demonstrates some of the ways a Tavistock or group-as-a-

---

* This section is based on a paper presented at the Ninth Scientific Meetings of the A.K. Rice Institute, Washington, D.C., 1989.

whole perspective can reveal opportunities for innovation and change in a sector that is routinely thought of as dealing with hopeless cases. The reader is probably familiar with the concept of projective identification. In reviewing this section, we invite you to consider what these abused, neglected children and their families as well as the systems which serve them represent or "hold" for all of us. (Note: In 1991, 1300 to 1400 children died as a result of physical abuse). We will present snapshots of our thinking, our work, and what we considered to be the relevant systems which impacted the care of these children.

A Texas Context

John Donne, who said, "No man is an island," did not hail from Texas. The state has a long legacy of rugged individualism. At the time the initial version of this paper was written, Texas ranked 49th in per capita expenditures for social services. In an era where children make up an increasing proportion of those in poverty, the implications for poor children and families are catastrophic. For example, as late as 1982, there were no publicly funded psychiatric beds for children and adolescents in the most populous county in Texas. Severely disturbed, indigent and lower middle class children were hospitalized in the forensic ward of the county general hospital. Only after reports that several children had been molested on this ward did a county judge order funding for two beds at a teaching hospital of the state medical school.

The Child Protective Service System in Texas is a joint responsibility of the state and the county. The state assumes responsibility to investigate cases of abuse and neglect and has the authority to remove children from their home if there is clear and present danger to the child. The county assumes responsibility to receive these children into custody and to care for them until they are returned home or safe alternative placements are found. The reader can imagine the ramifications of this split organizational structure, given the complexities of assuming custody of children.

In 1978, the county where the case study was located opened an emergency shelter for adolescents in protective custody. A state mental health clinic was established in the shelter facility to deliver evaluation and stabilizing treatment to the children. Such a shelter program was urgently needed, but the Child Protective Service System has been and continues to be poorly funded. The severe economic downturn which hit the Texas "oil patch" further depleted resources. Incidence of child abuse in Texas skyrocketed as funding for human services fell. The shelter's state funded mental health clinic was closed in 1984. The county approached the Child Mental Health Center (CMHC) discussed in the previous section for help in this crisis. A psychologist (CHI) with experience in the delivery of crisis services and the Tavistock approach was asked to organize a psychological services team at the Emergency Shelter with 1/4 of the funding that had been available to the state mental health clinic.

A colleague (UNI), at that time on the faculty of a local university, sought and was awarded a clinical training grant from the National Institute of Mental Health for the purpose of training future clinicians to address the lack of mental health services available to multi-problem, disadvantaged families with problem children and youth. UNI was then offered a position as consultant to the psychological services team being formed at the emergency shelter. Her consulting position evolved to include placement of NIMH-funded clinical students under her supervision on the team. An initial task for UNI thus involved the selection of a group of bright, motivated students with the intellectual and emotional capacity to tolerate the discovery that much of their academic training would not be applicable to providing services to underserved families. An initial task for the team was to form a working group that could define the inadequacies of its models and experiment with new ideas in this context. The following sections will describe some characteristics of the emergency shelter and the population it served as well as the team structures which evolved.

The Maltreated Children and Their Families

Below are presented excerpts of staffing notes from cases the team encountered in the first months of work at the shelter. These notes may help bring to mind the circumstances and characteristics of the children and the families they represent:

Melba (age 16). The shelter staff requested a consultation on a child who was acting in bizarre ways. The child said that she had been having nightmares where Freddy Krueger (of "Nightmare on Elm Street") was telling her to kill everyone in the shelter. When asked if anyone else in her family had a "strong temper," she replied that her father did and gave as an example an occasion where he nailed several of the family's pets to the walls of their home.

Charles (age 13). Charles was abandoned by his mother at a friend's home 9 years ago. Charles is now in the shelter because he allegedly sexually abused the friend's 16 year old retarded daughter.

Marissa (age 14). Resident was placed in custody last year. She is a chronic runaway, truant and a severe discipline problem at home and school. She is sexually promiscuous and drug involved. Parents have exhausted their insurance on outpatient and inpatient psychiatric hospitalization. She is well below average intelligence and residential programs in the area refuse to admit her.

David (age 13). Resident had been in custody for two years and in that time has gone through 30 placements. The last placement closed down. Tested IQ of 45. The previous night staff reported that he was running around nude.

Carol (age 13). She witnessed her mother being beaten to death by father. Child had tumors in both eyes and the surgery has left her face deformed. Child also alleged sexual abuse by her own father. Child was in placement at that time because she set up her grandparents' house to be burglarized by her boyfriend.

Augustina (age 14). Her father started having intercourse with her at age 7, and threatened to kill her if she became pregnant. Mother was aware of the situation. While the mother was pregnant, the father kicked her in the pelvic area. While the mother was hospitalized, the father had sex with child. After that incident, the child was admitted to the shelter and she had missed a period. There are six other children in the home. The family moved to the city from Mexico last year and no one in family has a green card.

Chris (age 15). He had become aggressive towards other shelter residents. The staff thought it was due to his impending discharge from the shelter. He had grown attached to the shelter staff and feared returning home.

A dramatic change in the types of children admitted to the shelter occurred in 1986 when radical cuts in funding resulted in the closing of state funded treatment facilities for emotionally disturbed children. This led to mass discharges from long term residential treatment programs of severely emotionally disturbed children in state custody back into their home communities. These children are extremely difficult to place in the remaining gamut of placement opportunities which are typically geared to take children with average IQ and no severe emotional disturbance (e.g., not violent, suicidal or psychotic).

The Shelter Organization

As mentioned earlier, a state mental health clinic had been operating in the shelter since its inception. This clinic had been closed abruptly due to funding cuts. The team was not warmly received by the shelter staff who had become attached to the state clinic's staff. The team had displaced their friends and we were regarded with suspicion and some animosity.

It quickly became clear that the shelter had very little in the way of organizational structures which would foster clarity of task for the staff, much less a sense of mutual support in the face of their awesome responsibilities and limited resources. The shelter is a 24 hour operation. Staff work in three 8 hour shifts. At the time we arrived there were no routine general staff meetings and no meetings of supervisory personnel. There was little or no communication and collaboration between shift personnel (e.g., reports to oncoming shifts on the status of residents or new arrivals were inconsistent at best). It was the colleagues' opinion that the children in the shelter were protected only by the personal authority and compassion of key staff members. The only cohesive force for these county employees seemed to be their collective defenses. For example, they would as a group project blame for the difficulty of their work onto the caseworkers who referred children into the shelter or onto the upper levels of management. The shelter staff would also ban together in group versions of fight-flight phenomena to escape the painful experiences generated by encounters with the children. Staff meetings would sometimes erupt in arguments or be filled with trivial banter about vacations.

The shelter accepted referrals from three community agencies: (a) state child protective service workers who referred children taken into custody due to severe abuse and neglect, (b) the county community youth service workers, who referred children in the midst of severe family crisis and/or dysfunction as manifested in truancy, poor school performance or pre-delinquent behavior, (c) juvenile probation officers who referred children arrested for delinquent, non-felony behavior as well as children in family crisis.

The physical plant and staffing patterns of the shelter, as well as its licensing guidelines were suitable for the provision of brief shelter to children (36 maximum) who presented no severe emotional, behavioral or physical abnormalities. The shelter ostensibly had control over which children were admitted but it was obvious that the county agency's executive director took it as a county mandate and responsibility to provide care for all children who would otherwise not receive care.

The shelter had no authority over the groups which admitted children to the shelter. If a child fell outside of the parameters for admission, the executive director would often override the shelter's decision to refuse admittance. Caseworkers from referring agencies would frequently delete important information about the child's background (e.g., recent attempts at suicide). These omissions may have been due to laziness on the part of caseworkers but it was more likely a strategy made necessary by the lack of any alternative placements for many of these children. This process was accelerated with the mass discharges of children in state custody from long term psychiatric treatment facilities back to the community and eventually back to the emergency shelter when all placement alternatives were exhausted or refused to take the child.

The majority of children admitted to the shelter came from families with chronic sexual and physical abuse. These children were mixed with children from families where unreported abuse may have occurred who had adopted a delinquent life style in reaction to their circumstances. New children were constantly added to the shelter population, often with incomplete information about their history and character. The opportunities for violence, abuse and other forms of acting-out among the children in the shelter were ubiquitous.

Evolved Team Structures

The two colleagues, CHI and UNI, were cognizant that their team was located at the intersection of several groups with varied missions and a history of antagonism. This included the various organizations that were represented within the team itself (e.g., a non-profit child mental health center, a state university, the National Institute of Mental Health). The Child Protective Service System itself was a composite organization. The structure which was supposed to reflect and promote the collaboration of state and county efforts clearly impaired authorization and accountability. The structure also seemed to facilitate projection of blame. It was also a demoralized agency ground down by the insatiable demands of the community's children and families, scapegoated by politicians and citizens, experiencing its own disillusionment and declining resources, suspiciousness and resistance to change. The work of forming and maintaining a team in this context in a way that satisfied CHI and UNI's eagerness to serve and their professional standards was immediately recognized as quite a challenge.

The team leaders, CHI and UNI, tried to develop a model for team structures that would be congruent with the various missions of the groups which interfaced at the shelter. They defined their principal mission as the delivery of first-class psychological services to the children who were served by the emergency shelter. Next they had to decide on what services were appropriate to the context. They held in mind that the basic task of the emergency shelter was to provide a safe environment for the children and assist in the transition from dangerous and/or neglectful situations to safer situations. The team's principal task was thus conceptualized as offering consultation and clinical services to assist the client (Child Protective Services) in its mission of serving the abused and neglected children served by the emergency shelter. The second task of training was conceptualized as offering opportunities to learn about the application of systemic thinking in community psychology. This opportunity was a true job on a clinical team with clear job description, task assignment, authority and accountability.

The extremely transient nature of the shelter population was another core factor that shaped the evolution of many team roles. All of the consultative and therapeutic roles on the team featured the notion that each contact should be a self-contained unit. The clinician could not count on seeing a child or family more than once. Children could be placed out of the shelter without notice, never to be seen by staff or our team members again. This was a major strain for the entire team and a unique factor that limited the application of more traditional clinical models.

The principal role of clinician was conceptualized as a consultant to the various groups that children are involved with through the sequence of pre-shelter setting, in-shelter and post-shelter placement. It was made clear to the clinician/trainees that their role held no authority over the children, their families or the state and county protective service workers. The team clinician's only authority was to offer and document their professional opinion as to what they thought about the dynamic situation at hand and to make recommendations when indicated as to what might be helpful. A prime example of this limitation in authority occurred whenever a crisis consultation revealed that a child was in danger of hurting her- or himself or others and the shelter staff did not agree that the circumstance warranted any immediate action.

The trainees struggled with doubts about their own competence, doubts about their prior training, and doubts about the treatability of the cases. These doubts frequently threatened to undermine quality service and creative problem solving. The team leaders found that constant examination of team member's collective and individual experience with a consistent questioning concerning how that experience might reflect the dilemmas and strains of their clients, be they children, parents or staff, was very useful in developing conceptual frameworks that held team members on track in their various roles. This process also facilitated team members' ability to offer useful interpretations to clients and their own team.

These principles were also employed in supervision. That is, within their roles as supervisors, UNI and CHI attempted to provide consultation rather than simple directions to the clinician/trainees. Each clinician had individual supervision in addition to two regular group supervisions. A weekly team meeting provided opportunities for team members to share information and attempt collective problem solving. A weekly didactic seminar in which brainstorming could occur at an intellectual level was offered along with live supervision of difficult cases. The request that trainees reflect on their role and their experience became the central question of supervision sessions and team meetings. It was a noteworthy clash of models which allowed the students to examine their institutional transference which was usually characterized by expectations that they were to have the knowledge, authority and responsibility to efficiently engineer change with clients.

The application of this principle of introspection included an analysis of the team's internal functioning as well as its interface with other agencies as an explicit agenda of supervision and training. Trainees read materials on federal, state, and community protective services mandates and deficiencies, and came to realize the true meaning of a systemic perspective and of the need to analyze levels and match intervention to the targeted level. For example, the team developed inter-agency workshops and staff groups that rechanneled frustrations with each other and the inadequacies of the larger system away from the youth and their families. These workshops appeared to make clinicians and youth workers less likely to scapegoat colleagues, themselves or the families for the constraints caused by the economic and political realities of the settings within which they worked.

Sample Interventions

The first major intervention emerged from the team's recognition that the basic contract requirement of providing psychological testing for purposes of placement was often unnecessary or actually functioned to expedite the unnecessary separation of children from their families. The team began requiring family evaluations before testing for placement in order to offer a more comprehensive evaluation of the children and their relevant social networks. This also helped to insure that children were not maintained in an unsafe family environment. The team also began to slowly offer more case consultation and family work with the objective of preventing unnecessary termination of parental rights.

The second intervention involved a shift from individually focused to group focused services for the children. Consistent with the mission of the shelter as a transitional facility, the team stopped offering individual therapy as a routine service and instead used a group format with the task of helping children reflect on the stresses they were experiencing in transition and their expectations for the future. The team maintained that the children's participation in any of our services was strictly voluntary. The shift to a consultative approach to group work was initially resisted by the children, shelter staff and by the team's own trainees. Introspection was certainly not modeled or reinforced in the coercive and neglectful families of these children. They had little or no previous experience with adults who truly attempted to help them put words to their distress. The trainees were continually pulled by a desire to be more directly helpful out of pity and/or the need to demonstrate their competence in the traditional role of behavioral and emotional modification.

Once the clinicians became better acquainted with the consultative model, the children demonstrated a surprising capacity to make use of the opportunity for introspection and support one another through the stress of transition. Some children could not be accommodated into the groups given their level of disorganization and the constraints on the group format (e.g., unpredictable membership). Those who gave clear evidence of their need for more structure were seen in individual sessions until they were stabilized or transferred out of the shelter. Individual consultation was also provided to children who presented as crises in the shelter (e.g., being physically threatening, noncompliant with minimum shelter rules, and/or unresponsive to typical shelter management strategies).

Clinicians also used the individual contact with the child as a data collection method and a gateway to offer consultation to the staff on if and how the child could be safely held in the shelter without being a danger to self or others. This issue was a continuing source of strain for the team and its members. That is, what to do in the situation where it was the team's opinion that the child could not be safely held in the shelter and the shelter staff did not agree. Team members had to be reminded frequently that the team had no authority over the Child Protective Service workers and that they were limited to giving and documenting their opinions. In essence, the team was reporting the situation of a child in danger to the child protective service system itself.

In terms of family work, the team developed a method of conceptualizing each session as a self-contained unit within a context of short-term, goal-oriented therapy and with an orientation toward pragmatic introspection, crisis management and system maintenance rather than long-term therapy with the ultimate goal of personality development. The team also focused on appreciation of the cultural diversity of the families (Korean, Vietnamese, Iranian, Haitian, as well as Mexican-American, Black-American and Anglo) and development of interventions that were not completely reliant on verbal exchange. The team leaders encouraged the application of techniques from many models as long as they fulfilled the goal of efficient, quality service.

As the shelter staff found the team's interventions to be relatively nonthreatening and in order for the shelter to be in compliance with licensing requirements, the county administration asked the team to provide a 24 hour on-call service to assist in the evaluation and management of crises. The team leaders proposed a system where representatives of the team would be positioned in two key meetings at the shelter: the intake staffing and the shift changes for the shelter. These particular meetings often included critical information that might allow the team to identify and obtain good background information on children who were likely to precipitate crisis situations in the shelter. It seems that in addition to affording opportunities to prevent or intervene early in crisis situations, the presence of team members at these meetings and the over-arching model of consultation shaped the way the shelter staff functioned even though clinicians would typically insert only a few comments or questions.

Another example of intervention focused on the group structure and dynamics of the shelter staff. It was obvious that there were serious splits between the shift supervisors and the upper management of the shelter. The team suggested that it might be helpful for the shift supervisors to have a routine meeting in which they could talk about the stresses and strains inherent in their role. The supervisors and shelter management agreed and a time was set. For the first months, most if not all of the supervisors would forget about the meeting time. The content and processes of the initial meetings appeared typical of groups with ineffective leadership (e.g., Bion's description of dependency and flight-fight basic assumption group processes). For example, the group would often have difficulty staying with the agreed upon task of discussing the stresses of their role. The group would instead talk about fantasy or recreational activities. At times, the group would bicker amongst themselves or complain bitterly about other sectors of the organization, the management, critical press, etc.

The directorship of the Emergency Shelter changed three times over the course of the first four years the team was on site. The most difficult aspect of consulting to this group was, of course, remaining on the task; the task of examining why the group could not work together to understand their experiences of working together in the agency. At one point near the end of the second director's tenure, the consultant to this group from the team (CHI) allowed himself to be pulled out of role and into providing covert management for the shelter operation under the guise of this consulting role. For example, the consultant found himself making numerous administrative suggestions including some which bore on specific shelter policies and even personnel decisions. The executive director of the child protective services at one point considered terminating the contract with CMHC in order to hire their own psychologist who would be accountable to the county. This reaction on the part of the Executive Director actually helped the consultant get back into his consulting role. CHI had been pulled (and leapt) over a boundary into shelter management activities for which he had no authorization. The threat of losing the contract vividly reminded CHI of the boundary and authorization of his role.

Over time, the shift supervisors were able to form a more cohesive working alliance and engage the director of the agency in helpful dialogue. They had previously been stuck in the view that their own director and executive director were not supportive of their efforts and scapegoated them for any difficulties that might arise (e.g., the executive director had a tendency to investigate his own personnel in a way that clearly conveyed an assumption of error on the part of his staff). It was recommended that the shelter supervisors request routine meetings with the executive director in order to enrich their relationships and reaffirm the linkage that they were working with and not against each other. Following the success of the consultation to the supervisors, a similar consulting role was requested for the line staff.

The team also designed interventions which focused on the intergroup dynamics between the various agencies involved in the children's lives. As mentioned earlier, the Child Protective Service is a joint state and county operation with closely linked responsibilities but two separate chains of authority. The comprehensive care of any child requires close coordination of the state and county systems which have distinct tasks and separate lines of authority. These separate task systems have to collaborate without the benefit of an overarching hierarchy of authority in order for the children's needs to be served. If any task falls between the two systems, then the child can suffer extended stays in temporary placements, go without needed medical attention, etc. As would be expected, those children who have the most special needs are the children who fall in the cracks between caretaking systems and are the ones who are most likely to be involved in crisis situations. The organizational split between the county and state systems compounded the difficulties inherent in the painful and awkward mission of assuming responsibility for derelict parents. The predictable effects of this organizational circumstance led to another type of intervention.

It was the team leader's hypothesis that the children and families import their stressful experience into the Child Protective Service systems where it is absorbed by the workers who then at times react with rejection and retaliation against the abused children and their families. Frustrated workers more typically attack their counterparts across the state/county boundary. To address this process the team proposed a set of meetings between state and county administrators to address the difficulties in collaboration across the boundary. The result was a workshop for state and county workers titled "The Consequences of Helping Hopeless Cases."

The format of the workshop included presentations by both state and county workers on what the stresses were in an ordinary day's work. The workers in attendance were then assigned to groups with equal numbers of state and county workers with a CMHC representative acting as consultant to the task. The task involved listening to a fictitious case that was a composite of the worst case client circumstances and characteristics. The workers were asked to discuss the stresses and strains of dealing with this sort of case in their role. Further, they were not permitted to discuss any problem solving strategies, only what was required of them, all the problems they might encounter and what this felt like. As might be predicted, the groups initially generated rapid-fire solutions to each scenario. With consultation, however, they soon were able to stick with the task of sharing the tedium, anger, demoralization and even horror of their daily work. In follow-up conversations and observations there was a substantial decline in overt and covert hostilities between state and county protective services workers as they interfaced at the shelter.

Outcomes

Because of the transitional nature of the setting, specific effects on the children are difficult to determine. To date the team has provided services to about 6000 children and families. There have been no suicides, homicides or rapes in the shelter. In a follow-up poll of children who participated in groups for sexually abused girls, approximately 30 percent of the respondents thought the group was of no use, 30 percent thought it was somewhat helpful and 30 percent thought their group experience was very helpful. This poll, taken on a sample of 30 children approximately 6 months after their stay in the shelter, compares favorably with most outpatient psychotherapy outcome research.

The most observable effects lie in the lasting changes in the organization of the shelter staff. In the opinion of the team leaders, the improved communication and clarity of roles and tasks is correlated with a clear reduction in the frequency of crises in the shelter population relative to the fluctuating level of emotional disturbance. The team has also observed an improved level of collaboration between the various agencies who interface in the emergency shelter. In terms of team services, requests for testings as a means of dealing with difficult cases stopped, family therapy is no longer fought, the shelter staff and case workers more routinely recognize and utilize team member's expertise as consultants and often ask team members to design continuing educational events for their staffs.

The size of contracts with the state and the county have steadily increased. The team has also trained over 70 graduate students in clinical psychology and related fields.

With respect to training, a rotation on such a team is difficult to market to prospective trainees. The idea of working with children who have been sexually and physically abused, families who are culturally diverse and indigent, within a system that is often the scapegoat for our society's own neglect does not present a pretty picture. Trainees ordinarily report that taking a role on this team is initially very stressful and confusing. They usually feel that the models they have been trained in do not apply to this job. There is often a related question of the actual impact of their work.

Trainees have reported that a major learning experience on the team is the experience of defining and maintaining a role of consultant to the children, parents and child-care professionals in the midst of very complicated circumstances. Over the course of the rotation, trainees ordinarily develop a heightened competence and a sense of confidence in their ability to formulate individual and systemic diagnoses along with pragmatic and dynamically informed interventions. In short, the rotation offers a unique opportunity for learning, sometimes painful, which challenges trainees to critically evaluate their clinical theories and assumptions about taking the role of a psychologist. Most of these say they plan to dedicate some portion of their career to underserved populations.

We conclude by returning to an earlier question—*what are these children and families holding for us all*, and a related question of responsibility. During periods of severe stress and crisis, the shelter staff often questioned who was truly responsible for the difficulties they faced in their work roles. The team members responded by offering the view that perhaps the children, the families or the upper levels of the Child Protective Services were not ultimately responsible. It was perhaps our own responsibility, the entire community, for failing to offer more support to these families. Who would want to care for the welfare of such children and families who embody what is considered pathetic, cruel, immoral and/or repulsive in human nature—who should? We hope that the reader will consider this question and consider also the possibility of contributing some of their valuable time and unique expertise in systemic thinking to these neglected children and families.

Revitalizing Human Service Organizations: An Action Research Perspective

Ellen Schall, JD
James Krantz, PhD

INTRODUCTION

The aim of this paper is to explore some central aspects in the attempt to revitalize organizations. The ideas we present concerning revitalization grow out of a large organizational change project aimed at revitalizing an urban human services organization, the New York City Department of Juvenile Justice (DJJ).

Revitalizing the moribund or stalemated organization requires replacing despair and resignation with hope and promise, establishing a unity of purpose and shared mission, and relating both the social and the technical systems realistically to the tasks. On the emotional side, the revitalized organization is one with newly found hope and excitement. The setting becomes a place where people can bring their creativity and enthusiasm for work instead of enacting the withdrawal and sense of sterility that pervades the stalemated organization. At the same time, revitalization requires careful organizational work and realistic development efforts; otherwise the hopes and dreams of members will be shattered. In other words, realistic and effective organizational structures must be designed

---

Ellen Schall is Martin Cherkasky Professor of Health Policy and Management, NYU, Robert F. Wagner Graduate School of Public Service, New York, NY. James Krantz, PhD, is affiliated with Gould, Krantz & White, New York, NY.

[Haworth co-indexing entry note]: "Revitalizing Human Service Organizations: An Action Research Perspective." Schall, Ellen, and James Krantz. Co-published simultaneously in *Residential Treatment for Children & Youth* (The Haworth Press, Inc.) Vol. 13, No. 1, 1995, pp. 55-74; and: *When Love Is Not Enough: The Management of Covert Dynamics in Organizations that Treat Children and Adolescents* (ed: Donna Piazza) The Haworth Press, Inc., 1995, pp. 55-74. Single or multiple copies of this article are available from The Haworth Document Delivery Service [1-800-342-9678, 9:00 a.m. - 5:00 p.m. (EST)].

and put into place if members have any chance of achieving their hopes for a revitalized setting.

In this paper, we review the underlying dynamics of human service organizations in general and those specific to organizations like DJJ and set the framework used to explore the issues with which we are concerned. Then we identify three distinct, though related, themes that illuminate important aspects of the revitalization process. The first involves the need for a strategic mission that resonates authentically with peoples' sense of their work and is capable of unifying the disparate parts of the organization around shared goals and purposes. The second concerns the tendency for grandiosity to emerge. How can leaders mobilize action, create hope and engage peoples' creativity without promoting excessively grandiose expectations and fantastic thinking? The third centers around questions of leadership and what kinds of leadership are required in different phases of revitalization. Finally, we offer several reflections that highlight some of the practical implications of our learning.

THE METHOD OF INQUIRY

Much of the thinking behind the change effort from which the insights in this paper are derived is the result of a collaboration between the organization's management and a small team of action researchers in the late 1980s. This paper represents part of that collaboration as well.

The approach to action research used by the consultants can best be described as "socio-analytic." This method is an open-systems approach that aims to understand an enterprise in its social, cultural, and economic contexts (Rogers, 1974). It does so through the application of several behavioral science conceptual lenses, including open systems thinking (Bertalanffy, 1956), psychoanalytic theory (Klein, 1948), Bion's (1961) theories of group development, and subsequent concepts which were developed as action researchers evolved this form of inquiry and intervention (Menzies, 1961; Jacques, 1955; Rice, 1963; Trist, 1951; and Miller & Rice, 1967).

Rather than basing change efforts on techniques or providing particular solutions to problems, the socio-analytic approach aims to help managers and staff develop an understanding of their internal and external environments and the tasks of their organization so that they develop greater insight and capacity to take up their roles. This involves developing an awareness of the typically unconscious forces which underlay work organizations and their performance in powerful ways.

The thinking in this paper represents insights that grew out of the inquiring relationship between the consultant/researcher and client system that is characteristic of action research (Clark, 1967). It is offered neither as a comprehensive overview of revitalization processes nor simply as a case study of a specific intervention. These ideas grew out of a socio-analytic consultancy aimed at assisting an organizational revitalization effort, and the ideas elaborated here point to directions for further research in the more general topic of revitalization.

THE UNDERLYING DYNAMICS OF HUMAN SERVICE ORGANIZATIONS

This section reviews, in more detail, key aspects of the conceptual framework used in this paper, particularly as they relate to human service organizations in general and to juvenile justice agencies in particular. Understanding the underlying dynamics of human service organizations such as DJJ requires a set of concepts that elucidates the unconscious dimensions of group life. This, of course, requires us to think about the irrational emotional underpinnings of collective life and the hidden assumptions and motives that often guide human behavior. Because our concern is with collective endeavor, the covert dynamics operating within and between groups are central. Approaching the system-as-a-whole as the unit of analysis, we have chosen a focus that renders visible the interaction between social process and the technical/structural aspects of organizational life.

Anti-task cultures. We take as a starting point for this review the work of Isabel Menzies (1961) on anti-task cultures. She describes the ways in which human service organizations, commonly asked to address enormously complex and difficult social problems with painfully few resources and little support, can too easily develop dysfunctional cultures. These dysfunctional cultures are usually characterized by very low morale, cynical attitudes of employees, emotional withdrawal by staff and ineffective task performance. The guilt and doubts inherent in such frustrating and troubling work, often exacerbated by poor quality performance, and the resentments generated by low quality of work life can be expressed in the form of anti-task cultures in which staff groups pursue gratifications and aims other than those derivable through working effectively. At their worst these anti-task cultures and the disruptive group dynamics can result in abuse of and violence towards clients. A less dramatic result, though perhaps no less destructive in the case of children, is inattention to children's needs.

Multiple and conflicting tasks. Menzies' analysis points to critical features underlying those human service organizations attempting to care for and change people that make them particularly susceptible to these forces. She also alerts us to the special challenges those managing these organizations must face to avoid the emergence of anti-task cultures. Specifically, the multiple and often conflicting mandates given these institutions (i.e., the tension between patient care and physician training in medical centers), amplified by the unrealistic expectations for impact and often inadequate resources to accomplish even modest outcomes, leads to a sense of failure with attendant doubts and anxieties.

These difficult tensions in organizational mission and strategy are particularly acute in juvenile correctional institutions because these institutions are expected to accomplish the security mandate simultaneously with the rehabilitation and caring functions. Fitch and Hewlings (1978) describe the ways in which these dual functions of control and care tend to promote fragmentation in correctional settings, with the functions split apart and lodged in different staff groups who are then likely to be in adversarial relations with one another.[1]

The impact of these often contradictory mandates is further complicated by the nature of the work itself in institutions that serve people. Staff in human service organizations are especially vulnerable to the strong emotional responses evoked by interaction with the clients with whom they work. Menzies (1979) illustrates the situation eloquently:

> The effect on staff of the human 'material' they work with is especially great in institutions whose clients are people in trouble. The clients are likely to evoke powerful and primitive feelings and fantasies in staff who suffer painful though not always acknowledged identifications with clients, intense reactions both positive and negative to them, pity for their plight, fear, possibly exaggerated, about their violence, or harsh, primitive, moral reactions to their delinquency. . . . The danger is that since the anxieties defended against are primitive and violent, defences will also be primitive. (p. 204)

Basic assumption life. Given the intense and often conflictual emotions stimulated by such work, and the frequent absence of institutional mechanisms for addressing them, it is hardly surprising to see groups within these institutions pursuing non-task aims. Anti-task cultures will typically be characterized by what Bion (1961) calls Basic Assumption groups. Bion's work on group emotionality and the way it either supports or conflicts with task performance provides an additional focus for understanding the way groups manage difficult and anxiety-producing situations on the unconscious level. Bion identified two groups always occurring simultaneously: the work group and the basic assumption group. His concept is a way of understanding two dimensions of all groups. The "work group" is systematically and scientifically pursuing its key tasks, while "basic assumption groups" are directed not to the achievement of the task per se but toward emotional gratification and emotional bonding. In work groups "the skills and interests of individual members are assessed rationally; role assignments are sensible; and individualized efforts are coordinated in a productive way" (Turquet, 1978, p. 356).

In contrast, basic assumption groups "offer simplifying constructions of reality and relatively uncomplicated leader and member roles" (Turquet, p. 356) which arise out of shared group fantasies. Important work-related anxieties are diminished and comforting emotional bonds created as groups turn to shared fantasies of an all-protective leader, group preservation through fight or flight, or the creative resolution of all tensions through the pairing of two members.

However, to think that work groups are "good" and basic assumptions groups "bad" misses Bion's crucial observation that both are necessary and simultaneous. Various emotional states complement–and are necessary for–certain tasks: appropriate dependency functioning in a hospital or flight emotions in a well-functioning army, for example. The key for effective work is to keep basic assumption life from overwhelming work group life, and for leadership to mobilize the particular quality of emotionality that will support rather than interfere with the task requirements of the moment (Rice, 1963).

Multiple tasks and basic assumption life. Involuntary total institutions pose particular challenges for leadership in this regard. The pursuit of each primary task establishes a constraint on what can be expected from the other (Miller & Rice, 1967); each task establishes emotional undertones that are often in conflict with one another. The requirements of accomplishing the dual tasks of caring for and detaining clients makes the articulation of a realistic mission both more difficult and more important. When leaders fail to provide this critical function of articulating a realistic double mission, their organizations are likely to be characterized by disruptions in group and inter-group relations, excessive basic assumption life, and ineffective performance.

Change and unconscious processes. Many of the anxieties and defensive patterns inherent in such difficult settings will render revitalization efforts all the more difficult and especially susceptible to being neutralized and distorted. Change is by itself anxiety-provoking (Jacques, 1955; Menzies, 1961; Miller, 1979; Alderfer & Brown, 1975). Change efforts in these kinds of organizations will inevitably be all the more difficult because of the high level of anxiety already present due to the tasks they are attempting to achieve.

THE SETTING

The New York City Department of Juvenile Justice provides detention, aftercare, and prevention services for juveniles in New York City. Most of the Agency's resources go to the detention function. The city mandate requires DJJ to detain children charged with crimes who are remanded by the courts pending the outcome of their cases. DJJ operates a secure detention facility,[2] Spofford, and a network of non-secure beds. The aftercare program grew out of the revitalization effort. Its purpose is to connect children released from detention with resources in their community in an effort to support children's successful return to their communities. The aftercare program, which is voluntary, emphasizes getting children back into school and helping them remain there. The aftercare work is part of the prevention function, which the Department attempts to achieve also through the range of program services provided children in detention, such as schooling, counseling, and medical care.

The Department was created as a separate agency in 1979. The system had become quite stalemated, characterized by unstable leadership at the midlevel with a high degree of turnover, fragmentation of mission, and little coordination between its various segments. Additionally, there had been a long-standing disconnection between the appointed leadership and the line staff.

Although there had been only one Commissioner from 1979 to 1982, there were five executive directors of the major facility, Spofford, during that same period. In the 28 years of Spofford's history there were 27 Directors. In contrast, 40% of the staff at Spofford had been there more than 20 years.

More importantly, and consistent with Fitch and Hewlings' (1978) thinking, there was virtually no connection between the secure and non-secure detention units, and within each unit the security and service functions were not coordinated and often in conflict. Staff's relationships with children were accordingly fragmented and there was a limited sense of overall goals for working productively with the children in detention.

Each part of the agency had its own distinct strengths as well as its difficulties. Spofford staff identified strongly with the children in their care and many were devoted to their well-being. Staff frequently reported they came to DJJ to give children the help they themselves had received from an important adult when they were young. On the other hand, Spofford had developed a very poor reputation and had received a lot of bad publicity both about escapes and the conditions under which children were held. In June 1978 the Mayor's Task Force on Spofford issued a report that referred to Spofford as a "case history in failure." Most troubling was the violence and abuse both staff to child and between children. Spofford thus exemplified many of the most disturbing features of anti-task cultures.

Working with deprived and extremely needy children, especially when identified with them, exacerbates one's own neediness (Menzies, 1979). At Spofford, staff members' identification with clients also heightened the pull to join and collude with the subculture that inevitably develops among institutionalized teenagers. Early on, the Spofford staff, when calculating the number of recipients of Christmas gifts to be donated by Yoko Ono, included themselves in the group.

Spofford as a bureaucracy was rigid and centralized, and the role dilemmas between custody and care had gotten drawn more sharply in recent years, with increasing emphasis on security. Although there were pockets of good individual work and a core of dedicated staff who cared a great deal about the children in custody, the staff's caring for children often seemed split from the large organization and "bootlegged."

Non-Secure Detention (NSD) was a less bureaucratic setting, at times to an extreme. It had few paper systems and little accountability. Its own manifestation of anti-task culture led it to emphasize the caring side of the mission, often to the severe detriment of the custody mission, as evidenced by a high abscond rate. NSD attempted to do a lot of work with children and some families, but the concrete services offered children in NSD (medical, mental health, education) were often of poorer quality than those offered in Spofford (though the Spofford services might become available to NSD residents once the sectors were seen as connected).

The Court Services unit had three major responsibilities: transporting juveniles from detention to the 15 court houses in five boroughs where children had to make court appearances; supervising children held in detention rooms in family court awaiting court appearances; and managing the admission process at Spofford. The unit provided a boundary function for the agency yet lacked a "consumer orientation." Basic Assumption life was rampant in the listless, disengaged quality of its culture. In flight from its task, the transportation division before 1983 had less than a 50% on-time delivery rate to court, which improved only after external pressure. Court Services was isolated from other units and, even within itself, was divided.

The headquarters office, "downtown," appeared to be an office in search of a purpose. The operating units saw it largely as irrelevant or as an impediment to their work and most useful as the place to lodge blame.

The top management staff defended itself against the difficulties of its work by taking as its main task from 1979 through 1982 the physical replacement of Spofford as if new borough-based facilities could magically fix all the problems. In doing so, it paid insufficient attention to the whole program, which suffered as a result.

Perhaps the trait "downtown" shared most with the operating units was a sense of impotence, of failure. It couldn't achieve its building agenda, and it was of little help to the operating units. While much of the work of headquarters is work on the external boundary, it did poorly there as well. There was little effective work with other city agencies, and DJJ had developed a reputation of being a difficult agency with which to work.

THE CHANGE EFFORT

The revitalization effort at the Department of Juvenile Justice had been going on at the time this was written for nearly six years.[3] The effort itself was multi-faceted, complex, and extensive. This paper reviews a portion of the first three years of this developmental effort. The work of the first phase involved creating the potential for serious change. This required assembling a management team and beginning to establish an administrative structure through which the new Commissioner could work. Part of the work in this period involved identifying the tendency to split apart the detention from the care or service elements of the Department, and to lodge aspects of them in different sectors of the organization. This tendency first had to be acknowledged and then overcome both in the organization as it evolved and in the Commissioner's own instincts, as she struggled with the need to see both custody and care as an essential part of each sector. In this beginning period considerable effort went into establishing an understanding of the Department's work and its culture.

The second phase of the change effort centered around the development of a strategic theme for the agency's change agenda, and the concurrent emergence of the tendency towards grandiosity and unrealistic thinking. Task forces were created, parallel to and apart from the standing lines of authority, to promote the discussion and thinking necessary to develop a long-range change effort.

Phase three rested on two bases. One was the attempt to ground the newly developed vision in a clearer sense of who the Department's clients were and what actually could be done with them. Second was the decision to tie more closely responsibility for the change agenda to the standing lines of authority, and in so doing attempt to foster more distributed leadership around the change initiative.

DEVELOPMENT OF A STRATEGIC THEME

Organizational metaphors and myths serve as unifying themes by which people internalize pictures of the work place and confer meaning on its various aspects (Dunphey, 1978; Smith and Simmons, 1983). These pictures in the mind shape the way in which people deploy their inner resources in relation to work–so they may see it as a place where they want to put their vitality or creativity or as a place where that is dangerous. In so many stalemated organizations, staff at all levels have internalized an image of the work place in which they bring only small parts of themselves to their work roles.

Producing a vision that mobilizes action requires the creation of metaphor that resonates deeply with people's experience and moves them to act in concert. Thus, the idea of "excellence" has been a catalyst for enormous innovation and change because it speaks to and mobilizes large numbers of people. Metaphors distill complex, interlocking problem situations so that actors may coalesce around a common guiding theme. These ideas, called *Ideas in Good Currency* by Donald Schon (1971), are an important element in transformational leadership.

Strategic themes are effective to the extent they not only resonate with people but allow them to validate and not disown their previous work (Gilmore & Schall, 1986). Grandiose, excessive or meaningless strategic programs may well promote heightened alienation or cynicism and invite increased disengagement from work.

Case management emerged as a strategic theme in two ways–it organized efforts to address operational problems and develop new projects, and secondly it served as a principle around which the organization was managed. Traditionally, case management refers to the way services in helping organizations are delivered to clients. The idea is that the array of services available are tailored specifically to the needs of each client. Case management has become "state of the art" in social service organizations (O'Conner, 1988) and there have been some recent experiments with this approach in juvenile post-adjudication correction facilities (Lindgren, 1984). Before DJJ, however, case management had never been attempted in a detention setting. Detention, where the clients' length of stay is unpredictable, often short and varies greatly depending on the trial process, had been seen as "dead time" where not much could be done for residents. While it must be remembered that many children stay in detention only a few days, another group stays for as long as a year or more. An important developmental period for these children was being overlooked.

As it developed in DJJ, case management involved providing a continuum of services to children from intake and assessment to the development of a service plan and the provision of services whether in detention or the community. To accomplish this the Department had to begin integrating previously fragmented services, having the needs of children, rather than the needs of the institution, drive service delivery and offering a coherence in the way the staff dealt with each child as he or she moved through different units.

Case management played a powerful role as a strategic theme in revitalizing DJJ. It resonated deeply with many staff's wishes to find a way of working effectively with children. But it was more than a metaphor; it was equally a way of organizing work and a principle for guiding change. It seemed to link the collective and individual levels simultaneously. While on the collective level it provided an overall idea of purpose with which people connected, it also guided task definition and work design on the unit level so that meaningful roles could be structured. In the attempt to shape and implement case management, roles were designed with which staff were able to engage and thus find a way in. In other words, the strategic theme also operated to reconfigure relationships between people and their work roles as well as inviting a more vital connectedness with the system.

By shaping the management system and the design of jobs, and by providing a guide for relating those to task, the strategic theme can harness basic assumption life to sophisticated work and diminish the prevalence of anti-task culture by linking people to their work more authentically.

THE DYNAMICS FOR HOPE AND GRANDIOSITY

Revitalization involves infusing a stalemated organization with new optimism. As necessary as that optimism is, it also contains the seeds of dysfunctional grandiosity. At its height in DJJ the grandiose thinking included the notion that the Department could "fix" kids, could establish an alternative high school system where children would succeed, could take over the work of other city agencies dealing with children, and could completely transform its own organization within a year. The delusional character of these dreams serve as illustrating the way Basic Assumption (Bion, 1961) group life can come to dominate the scene. In Bion's thinking, these grandiose hopes and wishes expressed group flight from frustrating realities.

The coming together of a group of people dedicated to humanizing the organization along with the strong mandate for change in DJJ often produced quite grandiose thinking. At times the thinking reflected assumptions of limitless resources, and was characterized by inattention to the realities of the existing organization, refusal to acknowledge limitations imposed by the wider environment, and fantasies of omnipotence. At an off-site planning retreat during the second year, the participants were asked to project five years into the future and describe what the agency would be like then. Many of the stories imagined DJJ outshining and capturing other agencies.

The grandiosity was "lodged"–or came to be expressed–primarily in certain individuals and units whose roles and tasks were well suited to it. In DJJ in the early years the planning unit as well as the Commissioner's office became, over time, the main locus of expansive thinking and at times grandiosity. While this was adaptive in the sense that it promoted hope and creativity, it had dysfunctional elements in that, for example, it disrupted the collaboration with the operational units. Line workers struggling to manage difficult children scarcely appreciated some of what they regarded as unrealistic ideas from downtown.

The co-mingling of helpful creativity and dysfunctional dreaming appeared within the strategy group, a structure designed to accomplish a key aspect of the development effort. This group, comprised of key managers and planning staff, was created by the Commissioner during the second phase of the change effort. She charged this group, which met monthly, with the task of developing a long-range strategic agenda for the agency, based on a central guiding theme of case management.

The Strategy Group's struggle to design case management in the Department exemplifies the ambiguous and often complex interplay of hopeful creativity and defensive grandiosity. For example, the group produced work plans that anticipated one month turn-around on tasks that ultimately took over a year to accomplish. In the group's more grandiose moments there was marked resistance to working with real information and grounded knowledge, and instead the group seemed in search of all-encompassing magical answers. To some extent the information needed to develop the program for children existed within the system. However, it was not brought together and developed in a way that it could be used. In a detention system children stay for varying and unpredictable lengths of time and planning for case management depended on a more detailed understanding of the population flows and, in particular, key indicators of length of stay. Designing a case management system to deliver individualized services depended on this kind of detailed knowledge.

The staff of the planning unit, charged with developing the data and proposing alternative designs, felt unable to complete these tasks for quite a long time. The unit maintained that the computer system was insufficient to develop the needed data base for the desired analyses. As became clear later, the capacity and necessary information were there. The unit's difficulty in accomplishing these tasks seems instead to represent a resistance to engaging in the concrete realties of implementing a case management system. The Basic Assumption functioning expressed a wish to remain with a "constraint-free" mode of planning.

Finally, when the Commissioner became able to insist on the delivery of this work, the planning unit produced it quickly and competently. The production of these documents unblocked the frustrated planning process and allowed several major decisions to be reached. Thus, a key shift occurred from unfettered visionary thinking to grounded, data-based planning for case management.

Several staff from the planning unit left in connection with this episode. The shift in orientation represented a loss to many members of the unit, some of whom were able to adapt and some of whom weren't. For example, one planner who most embodied the ideal of pure research, left to teach at a university in part as a result of this shift to the more grounded, applied concept of research which was required for the tasks DJJ faced.

Or, in another instance, despite a comprehensive review of the various ways case management had been implemented in other kinds of systems, the strategy group maintained that it lacked the necessary information to propose concrete designs for DJJ as if it could create a system free of the constraints and compromises inherent in other organizations' designs.

From these, and numerous other instances, a pattern emerged in which much of the hopeful creativity was expressed through the conceptualizing of case management, and much of the dysfunctional grandiosity was expressed in the difficulty of thinking realistically about its implementation. The dilemma faced by DJJ's management was how to encourage imaginative, innovative ideas and sensible, concrete approaches simultaneously. When the two were in alignment, development moved ahead. When Basic Assumption Life came to predominate in group thinking, imagination and hope tipped over into grandiose wishing and little progress could be made.

ISSUES OF LEADERSHIP

The ability to transmit a viable new mission, to get others to take leadership in developing and implementing the mission, and then in turn to mobilize others is a special capacity often thought of as charismatic leadership. Tichy and Ulrich (1984), for example, argue that revitalization requires this sort of "transformational leader," in Burn's (1978) sense. This view is probably overly "heroic" in placing hope for revitalization on the charisma or talent of a single individual.

A systems theory of leadership and change understands that leadership in organizations is a function of relationships, including those between formal leaders and followers (Miller & Rice, 1965). Roberts (1985), for example, has illustrated how the "charismatic phenomena" can result from a complex interplay of a varied set of factors. Her study suggests that the structural and contextual factors are more important than the particular qualities of an individual or the "authority of office" (Shils, 1969) in producing the "charismatic phenomena," although a strong leader is one important ingredient. In the case Roberts studies, the attribution of the special powers of charisma actually occurred after the leader's success and interestingly did not transfer with the leader to her next post.

Because leaders work through people (Spotts, 1976), the issues of group relations are very closely related to those of leadership. Often people other than the formal leaders provide the decisive leadership in work groups, and groups go in directions other than those the "leader" mandates. Ultimately the direction work groups go depends upon the complex web of implicit relations that comprise the group. Formally designated leaders inevitably shape and influence these relationships, though they are also affected and shaped themselves by the organization's culture and its group processes.

While revitalization is often credited to the presence of a charismatic leader, we hypothesize instead that the charismatic phenomena is but one phase of revitalization. Our experience suggests that organizations undergoing change require different forms of leadership at different points and that charismatic leadership can serve as a transitional phase in enabling an organization to "unfreeze" its long-standing patterns while searching for new approaches, but is dysfunctional in the long-run. The dependency on the charismatic figure must be relinquished in favor of more shared leadership if change efforts are to be institutionalized and continuity achieved.

Miller (1979) suggests the need for a "dependency receptacle" in change efforts. This stems from the fact that the institutionalized modes of operating–the structures, policies, customs, etc.–that are being reshaped are also being used by members to reinforce their defenses against painful anxieties (Menzies, 1960; Jacques, 1955). As structures and methods of operation are changed, members need a repository for their dislodged dependency and anxieties. Leaders need to fulfill that function until new patterns and structures are in place, patterns which will again simultaneously help members defend themselves against work-related anxieties and enable the enterprise to work effectively. The attribution of charisma to leaders at this moment can be understood as an expression of the work group's need for such a repository, and the emergence of the charismatic phenomena as an important transitional moment in the revitalization process. The presence of a leader who can fulfill those needs and expectations at the moment is therefore an important factor in revitalization. In Bion's terms, Basic Assumption dependency culture may be a necessary emotional underpinning to successful transitional phases.

DJJ went through its own version of a charismatic phase around the Commissioner, who for a time was regarded as the source of all creativity and authority. These dynamics can be seen in the way DJJ created and used the strategy group. It was created by the Commissioner as a forum parallel to the existing administrative structure in an attempt to "unfreeze" the organization. Its design aimed at generating the most creative thinking possible in developing the new mission, and in doing so, brought together key actors in the system from across several hierarchical levels all working directly with the Commissioner. This approach succeeded in generating many good ideas and a lot of energy. It established strong cross-unit development work, and perhaps most importantly, served to diffuse the vision of case management throughout the top managers.

On the emotional level, it allowed and reinforced dependency on the Commissioner. The strategy group fostered the view that she, and she alone, could authorize new ideas. As a result, it de-emphasized issues of delegation, authorization, and representation. These issues became more central to the change process as the effort shifted from developing ideas and articulating a new vision to implementing case management. Thus, while serving important task-related functions, the strategy group also came to reinforce the organization's dependency on its leader and other members' longing for her to be the source of all change and decision making.

In attempting to manage this, and move the agency ahead, the Commissioner decided to dissolve the strategy group and create a new set of forums that corresponded structurally to the actual administrative hierarchy. She created two new top level groups charged with carrying on the cross-unit, department-wide aspects of the change initiative, and integrating the changes into the on-going operations. In addition, each unit continued with its own decentralized work.

This shift marked an important moment in the agency's development and in the change effort as well. The decision to invest the standing lines of authority with responsibility for carrying the change ahead signalled a move from reliance on charismatic leadership to a phase of shared leadership. This, in turn, potentiated new sources of energy and empowered a wider range of people to contribute to the development of a case management agenda.

The meaning of leadership and the appropriate behavior of leaders evolved over time as the organization changed. This is consistent with research findings which point to the need for a matching of leadership style with organizational life cycle (e.g., Kimberly et al., 1980; or Tichy and Ulrich, 1984). The experience at DJJ suggests two things: (1) that as a revitalizing mission diffuses through the organization, decentralization of leadership must accompany it to prevent the emergence of disabling dependency on the top managers; (2) leaders need to be able to grow and adapt along with their organizations.

IMPLICATIONS FOR MANAGERS

In this section we offer a set of reflections drawn from the kinds of experiences we detailed in the preceding sections. We distill these reflections into three key learnings that grow out of this long-term revitalization effort which we regard as having practical importance for managers. They concern the importance of investing in the organization; developing a reflective capacity in the organization; and taking the irrational and unconscious aspects of the organization seriously.

Investing in the organization. Revitalization goes beyond specific program initiatives and is about change in the very fabric of the organization. Our hypothesis is that one must invest in the organization in order to revitalize it. This involves finding the organization's strengths and building on them, and inevitably entails long-term slow, patient work. Investing in the organization is a stance that takes seriously the organization's capacity to do its fundamental work. This then entails a primary focus on the foundations of the organization: its culture, structure, reward systems, patterns of communication, values and mission.

For purposes of illustration we contrast this approach to more typical change efforts that involve a select number of high visibility projects aimed at producing short-term results. Commonly an administration is in place for two to three years and its horizon is geared to such efforts which are typically staff driven, *ad hoc* additions to the organization's structure rather than an integral part of its operations, and are based on a view of the organization as standing in the way of what the executive wants to accomplish. In contrast, long-term revitalization efforts, we suggest, have the following attributes:

- A mission rather than program orientation.
- Stress on development of the standing organization's capacities.
- Focus on "small wins" (Weick, 1984), with an understanding that the first wins will be important internally but of little significance to the outside world.
- Taking the organization's chain of command and role relations seriously.
- Seeing the organization as the instrument of achieving change rather than as a barrier to change.
- Leadership that is collective and shared; it being neither heroic nor adversarial, operating against the organization.

By definition, revitalization begins with a stalemated situation. Therefore, there is no requirement that the organization be in good shape before this kind of work can begin. Because systems have enormous inertia and are extremely slow to change in deep ways, or are dynamically conservative in Schon's terms (1971), however, this kind of work does require time. Thus investing in the organization entails both a different stance toward the organization and a longer term time commitment from the top.

> *Development of a reflective capacity.* Just as investing in the organization implies a certain stance toward organizational change, the development of a reflective capacity is one in which people at all levels can think about what they are doing, link their thoughts and feelings in the service of learning about the organization, and then use their learning in the way they manage themselves in their roles. Unlike Basic Assumption groups which have no time, tolerance, or sympathy for thinking (Turquet, 1978), the sophisticated work required to revitalize an organization requires a commitment to dialogue, thinking, and introspection.

This reflective capacity involves an interpretive stance toward one's experience in an organization. From this perspective one hears anecdotes not as facts but as clues and sees one's own experience as yielding information about the larger social system. This allows people to develop hypotheses, act, and make mid-course corrections as the learning continues. "Learning as one goes" inevitably precludes a master work-plan approach which, while comforting, interferes with the opportunity to learn from the unexpected.

This is an anxiety-confronting rather than anxiety-evading approach. In acknowledging and confronting work-related anxieties, members have greater personal resources available for working, in part because the feelings and the conflicts underlying these anxieties are no longer being denied and projected and in part because the energies used to defend against troubling aspects of organizational life are then freed for other purposes. The intense anxieties associated both with change and with the work of human service organizations (Menzies, 1979; Alderfer & Brown, 1975; Trist, 1974; Miller & Gwynne, 1972) render the reflective stance painful, yet ever the more important.

As with any task, the necessary conditions must be present. In this case, that involves both time set aside at least specifically for reflection and a structure suitable to support this kind of work. In DJJ, both the Strategy Group and Executive Staff were such forums. The Executive Staff set aside half of its weekly two-hour meeting to discuss the question "What is going on in the organization from which we can learn?" As the group explored this question many of the implicit dynamics influencing the organization were enacted in the Executive Staff. Having a consultant present who was able to help the group interpret and learn from what was going on was particularly helpful.

> *Taking the irrational and the unconscious seriously.* The unconscious, irrational dimensions are both the source of destructiveness as well as creativity in group and organizational life (Hirschhorn, 1988; Krantz, 1987). Change, in and of itself, releases powerful feelings. And revitalization requires people to bring their feelings, their creativity, and their passions to their work to a far greater degree than in stalemated organizations. This creates a richer and more complex affective field in the organization which offers the potential for either enormous growth and development or chaos and destructiveness. Thus, attention to the irrational aspects of shared work life becomes both more productive and more important under these conditions.

Equally, appreciation of these aspects of organizational life serves as a rich and powerful source of data about the organization. Without an appreciation of this strata of organizational life, it is unlikely that the resistances to change can be understood nor can the group's forces for change be realized (Smith and Berg, 1987).

For example, the ability to develop a program that linked custody and care in DJJ was able to proceed only after the Executive Staff acknowledged their feelings first about being jailers and second about locking up minority children. Also, in such a diverse and multicultural setting as DJJ, the ability to explore the difficulties of working across race, gender, age, and class boundaries also enabled more sophisticated, task-oriented collaboration.

The exploration of the irrational and unconscious began at the top. It became clear that once difficult issues, particularly those which involved the way intergroup relations amongst racial, gender, ethnic, age, and hierarchical groups effected DJJ's work, were acknowledged at the top levels, the next levels of the organization were freed up to explore the issues as well. The ability to engage sectors and units in a task-related exploration of these issues emerged as an important leadership capacity at DJJ as the organization became more able to tolerate working explicitly with its own unconscious processes.

CONCLUSION

Human service organizations are faced with an ever greater need to respond to distressed elements in society. Increasingly, these organizations are confronting the need to find the sort of frame-breaking changes (Tushman et al., 1986) which can reverse the chronic burnout and alienation of staff. On the basis of an action research effort at New York's Department of Juvenile Justice we have attempted to illustrate some of the underlying dimensions of revitalizing human service organizations. To be sure, every revitalization or renewal effort will be different in that it will respond to a unique set of local conditions, actors, and challenges. At the same time, our experience points to some potentially common elements in human service organizations that may illuminate other efforts to revitalize stalemated settings.

NOTES

1. This is particularly damaging for children in custody. To the extent that these institutions are charged with helping the children they are detaining, it is crucial that staff achieve fully mature authority relations with the children, requiring staff to combine both the control and caring aspects. "The management of delinquents has to demonstrate not only that authority represents both control and concern but that control and concern are indivisible attributes of any management." (p. 246)

2. In a secure facility children's movement is generally restricted. Secure facilities are characterized by the presence of bars on windows, locked doors and fences. Non-secure facilities, generally group homes and foster homes, are characterized by the absence of such hardware and allow for children to be more a part of the local community.

3. Since undertaking its efforts, DJJ has made major strides toward revitalizing itself and putting a quality case management system in place for its children. Though work remains to be done, the program has received a great deal of recognition, including a Ford Foundation/Kennedy School of Government "Innovations" award for one of the ten outstanding innovations in city and state government in 1986. Although it is not within the scope of this paper, it may be of interest to point out that many of the indices of stalemate or dysfunction have been reversed and there is a great deal of evidence pointing to the success of this revitalization effort which has been accomplished without a substantial increase in expenditure.

REFERENCES

Alderfer, C. and Brown, D. *Learning from Changing*. Beverly Hills, CA: Sage Publications, 1975.

Bertalanffy, L. *General Systems Theory*, General Systems, 1:1-10. 1956.

Bion, W.R. *Experience in Groups*. New York: Basic Books, 1961.

Burns, J. *Leadership*. New York: John Wiley & Sons, 1978.

Clark, A. (ed.) *Experimenting with Organizational Life*. New York: Plenum Press, 1976.

Dunphey, D. "Phases, Roles, and Myths in Self Analytic Groups" in *Analysis of Groups*, G. Gobbord, S. Hartman & Mann, eds. San Francisco: Jossey-Bass, Publishers, 1978.

Fitch, J.H. and Hewlings, D.G. "Organization and Training for the Task of Treatment in the Prison Service," in E. Miller (ed.) *Task and Organization*. New York: Wiley & Sons, 1978.

Gilmore, T. and Schall, E. "Use of Case Management as a Revitalizing Theme in a Juvenile Justice Agency," *Public Administration Review*, May/June 1986, pp. 267-274.

Hirschhorn, L. *The Psychodynamics of Work*. Boston, MA. MIT Press, 1988.

Jacques, E. "Social Systems as a Defence against Persecutory and Depressive Anxiety." In *New Direction in Psycho-Analysis*. London: Tavistock Publications, 1955.

Kimberly, J., Miles, R. and Assoc. *The Organizational Life Cycle*. San Francisco: Jossey-Bass Publishers, 1980.

Kimberly, J. and Quinn, R. *Managing Organizational Transitions*. Homewood, Ill.: Richard D. Irwin, Inc., 1984.

Klein, M. *Contributions to Psycho-Analysis 1921-1945*. London: The Hogarth Press, 1948.

Krantz, J. (ed.) *Irrationality in Social and Organizational Life*. Washington, D.C.: A.K. Rice Institute, 1987.

Lawrence, P. and Dyer, W. *Renewing American Industry*. New York: The Free Press, 1983.

Lindgren, J. "Continuous Case Management with Violent Juvenile Offenders," in R. Mathias (ed.) *Violent Juvenile Offenders*. San Francisco: NCCD, 1984.

Menzies, I. "Staff Support Systems: Task and Anti-Task in Adolescent Institutions," in Hinshelwood & Manning, eds. *Therapeutic Communities*. London: Routledge & Kegan Paul, 1979.

Menzies, I. "The Functioning of Social Systems as a Defense Against Anxiety." *Human Relations 13*, pp. 95-121, 1961.

Miller, E.J. and Rice, A.K. *Systems of Organization*. London: Tavistock Publications, 1967.

Miller, E. "Autonomy, Dependency and Organizational Change," in Towall, D. & Harris, C. (eds), *Innovation in Patient Care*. London: Croon Helm, Lts.: 1979.

Miller, E. and Gwynne, G. *A Life Apart*. London: Tavistock Publications, 1972.

O'Conner, G. "Case Management System and Practice," in *Social Casework: The Journal of Contemporary Social Work*. February (1988) pp. 97-106.

Rice, A.K. *The Enterprise and its Environment*. London: Tavistock Publications, 1963.

Roberts, N. "Transforming Leadership. A Process of Collective Action," *Human Relations*. Vol. 38, No. 11, pp. 1023-1046. 1985.

Rogers, K. "The Socio-Analytic Approach to Organizational Consulting." (unpublished, 1974).

Schon, D. *Beyond the Stable State*. New York: Norton, 1971.

Shils, E. "Center and Periphery." In *The Logic of Personal Knowledge: Essays in Honour of Michael Polanvi*. Glencoe, Ill.: The Free Press, 1961, pp. 117-120.

Smith, K. and Berg, D. *Paradoxes of Group Life*. San Francisco: Jossey-Bass Pubs., Inc. 1987.

Smith, K. and Simmons, V. "A Rumpelstiltskin Organization: Metaphors on Metaphors in Field Research." *Administrative Science Quarterly*, 28, pp. 377-392. 1983.

Spotts, J. "The Problem of Leadership: A Look at Some Recent Findings of Behavioral Science Research," In Lassey, R. & Fernandez, R. (eds.) *Leadership and Social Change*. La Jolla, Ca: University Associates, 1976.

Tichy, N. and Ulrich, D. "Revitalizing Organizations: The Leadership Role," in John Kimberly and Robert Quinn (eds.) *Managing Organizational Transitions*. Homewood, Ill.: Richard D. Irwin, Inc., 1984.

Trist, E. "Resistance to Innovation," paper presented to the Innovation Canada Seminar, 1974.

Trist, E. & Bramforth, K. "Some Social and Psychological Consequences of Coal-getting," *Human Relations*, Vol. 4, No. 1. 1951.

Turquet, P. "Leadership. The Individual and the Group" in Gibbard, G., Hartsman, J. & Mann, R. eds. *Analysis of Groups*. San Francisco: Jossey-Bass, Publishers, 1978.

Tushman, M., Newman, W. and Romanelli. "Consequence and Upheaval. Managing the Unsteady Pace of Organizational Evolution." *California Management Review*. Vol. 29, No. 1, 1986.

Weick, K.E. "Small Wins. Redesigning the Scale of Social Problems." *American Psychologist*. Vol. 9, Jan. 1984, pp. 40-49.

The School Romance:
Approaches to the Subjective Experience
of School Life

Daniel B. Frank, PhD
Dennis L. McCaughan, PhD

Perhaps the greatest of all pedagogical fallacies is the notion that a person learns only the particular thing he is studying at the time.

–John Dewey

SUMMARY. This paper aims to map the emotional landscape of school life through stories that illuminate the psychodynamics of idealization, disillusionment and reparation.[1] Schools are complex social organizations that can be better served when educators are able to inform their practice with a comprehensive understanding of how its various constituents–students, teachers, parents, administrators–relate to each other and strive to make sense of their varied sub-

Daniel B. Frank, PhD, is Head of the Upper School at the Francis W. Parker School in Chicago. He is also Lecturer in the Department of Psychiatry at the University of Chicago, Lecturer in the School of Education at DePaul University, and on the Human Development and Learning Faculty of the Institute for Psychoanalysis. Dennis L. McCaughan, PhD, is in private practice and is Clinical Assistant Professor of Psychology in Psychiatry at the University of Illinois at Chicago.

[Haworth co-indexing entry note]: "The School Romance: Approaches to the Subjective Experience of School Life." Frank, Daniel B., and Dennis L. McCaughan. Co-published simultaneously in *Residential Treatment for Children & Youth* (The Haworth Press, Inc.) Vol. 13, No. 1, 1995, pp. 75-105; and: *When Love Is Not Enough: The Management of Covert Dynamics in Organizations that Treat Children and Adolescents* (ed: Donna Piazza) The Haworth Press, Inc., 1995, pp. 75-105. Single or multiple copies of this article are available from The Haworth Document Delivery Service [1-800-342-9678, 9:00 a.m. - 5:00 p.m. (EST)].

75

jective experiences of the school. Current school experience is influenced by longstanding and complex identifications with prior school and family experiences. We call this highly personal identification with the school and the enduring influence of memories of the school on our current perceptions, *the school romance. [Article copies available from The Haworth Document Delivery Service: 1-800-342-9678.]*

DESPERATELY SEEKING SCHOOL AND THE CONTRADICTIONS OF SCHOOL LIFE

The school is an essential institution in our culture. No other social organization shares with parents as much responsibility for the growth and development of young people. Understanding our society's relationship to the school and the many expectations we have of school life is important to further our understanding of the subjective experience of school life. This inquiry, however, needs to be understood in the context of the rapidly changing world in which we live.

Many find the pace and degree of current social change turbulent, chaotic, indeed, overwhelming. Adults and children struggle with feelings of estrangement and disconnection as they search for a sense of meaning and coherence in their lives. In the context of a tough economy and a fractured culture, parents and children try desperately to balance their feelings of uncertainty with their hopes and dreams for the future. As other social institutions–the family, the church, the neighborhood community–struggle in their capacities to help parents raise and educate children, there is increasing pressure for schools to be the one stable and secure place where children can learn and grow.

More and more parents, policy makers and educators are looking to the school to heal in children, and in themselves, psychological wounds resulting from our society's struggle to cope with change, loss and disillusionment. More and more, the school is pressed to provide young people educational opportunities that will allow them to develop a sense of coherence and self-esteem, and to convey to students–and to their parents–the core values of our culture. In places where entrenched poverty, random violence and systematic repression assault children's aspirations, the school, in the eyes of many parents, teachers and students both oppresses the powerless and at the same time also perseveres as a symbol of possibility, hope and reparation over injuries committed to the human spirit. Even in the best of schools, where students are eager to learn, where adults have provided students and their teachers with the best of educational resources, the school can remain a complex, even confusing and ambivalent, symbol of hope and hostility, dreams and disappointment, optimal and arrested development.

Schools are curious and wonderful places, largely because of their multiple and complex roles and functions. Schools are institutions designed to develop reason yet they are also social organizations structured with subtle and stunning contradictions. These tensions are both social and psychological, both culturally shared and deeply personal. The school aims to focus teacher and student attention long enough so that ideas and information can be assessed in safe classrooms and in a steady and reliable manner, all while the school has become more and more the object of almost unbearable public anxiety about the present and future of American life. The school strives to develop the common good as well as enhance the personal experience of each individual student. The school is designed to support the growth of young people, as it also aims to support the needs, ideals and values of adults who inevitably have different, even competing, points of view from one another. Aimed at preparing young people for the future, adults who administer and teach in schools often defend with force the sanctity of tradition. Devoted to the development of reflection and understanding, the school is also a powerful object and source of great conflict, passion and desire for children and adults across the life course. Founded on enlightenment conceptions of character development, creative excellence and civic pride, schools struggle regularly with the tough, seamier realities of tight budgets, multiple institutional expectations and competing constituent agendas and world views.

Children and adults look to the school to provide them with more than just an education. The school stands as a symbol and a structure that can heal injuries, repair damage, right past wrongs. The experience of school life is indeed closely connected with our experience of American life. Americans expect the school to provide students with an education that will equip them with concrete, identifiable opportunities for success and prosperity–the promise of American life. Americans also live with a disquieting fear, even envy, that the educational system will disappoint them, that their dreams will be thwarted, that the school will remind them of what they might lose, have already lost, or may never have. Schools struggle constantly with the tensions of multiple aims. Reason and passion collide as schools search to find ways to narrow the gap between their ideals and the realities they confront. The world of the school is shaped both by the external realities of politics, finances and values and by the internal fantasies and private emotional responses of students, parents and educators. Whether day or boarding, private or public, comprehensive or residential treatment, the school is a site where reality and fantasy meet.

Somewhere between the clarity of a school's publicly stated mission and the actuality of how its daily practices and processes are experienced by individuals and groups within the school, lies the phenomenon we are calling *the school romance.*

THE SCHOOL ROMANCE:
A PARADIGM FOR UNDERSTANDING
THE SUBJECTIVE EXPERIENCE OF THE SCHOOL

The concept of *the school romance* reflects Freud's story about the family expressed in his 1908 paper, "The Family Romance." Freud discussed how a child's fantasies about his or her parents are shaped by the pleasures and disappointments of family life. He stated: "The freeing of an individual, as he grows up, from the authority of his parents is one of the most necessary though one of the most painful results brought about by the course of development" (1908:237). The child, he argued, having initially conceived of his parents as gods, inevitably goes through a period of disillusionment. In this process, the child, in fantasy, replaces his actual parents with idealized parents who occupy a higher social station and who command more prestige. These fantasies are often set in motion (often in reference to a "rival" brother or sister) when the child feels slighted or momentarily unloved. Although expressive of hostility and a sense of injury, these efforts at replacement are really an expression of the child's deep attachment. Freud (1908:240-241) writes:

> Indeed the whole effort at replacing the real father by a superior one is only an expression of the child's longing for the happy, vanished days when his father seemed to him the noblest and strongest of men and his mother the dearest and loveliest of women. He is turning away from the father whom he knows today to the father in whom he believed in the earlier years of his childhood; and his phantasy is no more than the expression of a regret that those happy days are gone. Thus in these phantasies the overvaluation that characterizes a child's earliest years comes into its own again.

Freud recognized that fantasy and illusion serve to protect the psyche from the inevitable experience of disappointment and loss. The fantasy is a form of nostalgia reflecting the mourning of the past and the limitations of the future.

The structure of *the school romance* can be understood as parallel to

Freud's family fantasy. The school, next to the family, is the most important institution of childhood. Our vulnerability as children is widely acknowledged and accounts for part of Freud's emphasis on fantasy as a means for the regulation of self-esteem. Psychoanalysis has documented the ways in which we attempt to regulate our experience through the use of fantasy and to master that experience through the organization of an inner world of persons, ideals and events powerfully linked with affect.

In *the school romance*, the school becomes the object of fantasies reflecting aspects of family life as well as those influenced by the challenges of school life itself. Each of us develops a subjective–at times unconscious–set of attitudes towards school. These attitudes, expressive of conflict and potential, come to life during the course of the school year as students, teachers, parents and administrators respond to the routines, rituals and developmental challenges that school requires (Salzberger-Wittenberg, Henry and Osborne, 1983). At times, conflicts between parents and teachers and teachers and students reflect the contradictory nature of our emotional responses to the school. We have all been to school and we each have our own personal responses to our respective school experiences. Yet, our consciously held views are often at odds with the more emotionally laden experience of *the school romance* where parents and teachers alike bring with them to current school situations their own fantasies and associations to past school experiences.

We might, for example, share a common observation of a student at a desk or a teacher at a blackboard but we each will have a personal set of associations and memories to those common images, ones based on our own past experiences. As time passes, and our actual school days recede into the past, we tend to forget the everyday, mundane aspects of our school experience. Instead, we tend to remember with more clarity those moments of emotional significance: the mastery of a difficult problem; the exhilaration of social or athletic accomplishment; the sick feeling of failure; the special reward of recognition; the indifference of certain teachers and the kindness of others. Adults and children bring to their current school experiences salient emotional aspects of past relationships in school and at home. Parents indeed bring more than their children to school, and teachers and administrators bring more to work than their briefcases. Each is accompanied by memories and associations to his or her own childhood school and family experiences.

These memories and fantasies include feelings of longing and revenge, the desire for reparation and mastery over past psychological wounds. They also can include a desire for immortality through reliving what now seems like once simpler days, now long gone, to the complexities of adult life and the middle-age realization that, as adults, we have probably already lived most of our lives. These memories and associations can, unwittingly, influence the here-and-now formation of positive alliances with others in school.

For most children, the school stands midway between home and community, midway between the presence of parents and the wider public world. For them, the school serves as a potential transitional space between a child's experience of parental values and expectations and the child's own emerging sense of the values and expectations held by his or her society. In this transitional space, the school can facilitate a child's emotional growth and cognitive development by providing policy, program, personnel and philosophy that can provide an appropriate developmental structure and texture to promote a child's experience of learning.

At the core of a child's capacity to learn is his experience of developing both a sense of separateness as an individual and as a connected member of an interdependent group. Like other formative experience that has its origins in the family, school experience becomes an integral part of the self. This experience of the school–*the school romance*–is shaped by both the reality of school life and by the child's effort–through the use of fantasy–to manage the inevitable injuries to the sense of self that the school engenders. The very process of learning is not without anxiety. In order to learn we inevitably risk pride and shame for fear of being found wanting and insufficient, and thus being rejected. To learn in school, students must open themselves up to the reality that they are in need of acquiring knowledge and understanding from others. This process can make students feel vulnerable, inadequate, disillusioned and injured. And this dynamic parallels a common wish and ideal held by students, teachers and parents that students will be able to learn in an atmosphere that will make them feel good about themselves, their accomplishments and provide them with continuous experiences of respect, recognition and integration (Fuqua, 1993).

The meanings these relationships have for us are organized in the symbolic images represented in our memories and associations and in the narrative structure of the stories we tell ourselves and others about our lives. That school should have such an impact on our lives is hardly surprising. We have all been to school. And, for most children, only the family has played a more important role in the development of a child's life. In this sense, the authority of the teacher and the school is consonant with parental authority, and our disillusionment with the school is not unlike that with our parents. We hope for so much and wish that our teachers and our school would forever be as we once believed we experienced them. As one writer notes, the ambivalence students can feel toward their teachers can be profound:

> We loved them, or hated them, or even despised them, but never escaped their daily presence in our thoughts. What is it about teachers that affects us so? What is it about teachers that gives rise to such powerful reactions, such vigorous emotions? What is it that causes us to identify teachers as such lasting, vital, irreplaceable influences in our lives? Surely some strange power is at work. And that power may remain forever shrouded in mystery, forever resistant to precise description. But it's there. We feel its presence. We know its permanence. It is for this that we love our teachers or hate them, but are unable to forget them.[2]

The writer cited above notes that students can *either* love *or* hate their teachers. We would add, however, that the same teacher who is the object of great affection and respect *also can be at the same time* the object of hate and hostility. The nature of ambivalence and the mark of its developmental significance is that a person can maintain simultaneously multiple and contradictory feelings about oneself and/or another person. Maintaining multiple feelings toward another without regressing into a stance where it is necessary to separate and isolate one's feelings can promote growth by inhibiting our human tendency to disavow painful aspects of our experience. In other words, the beloved teacher can also be the same teacher in the children's song: "... throw the teacher overboard and listen to her scream."

TRANSFERENCE TO THE SCHOOL

Similar to the ambivalent ways children experience their parents, the dynamics of ambivalence also characterize the ways in which students, teachers and parents experience their relationships with each other. Once again, Freud himself offers us a rich example of what we are calling *the school romance*. In an essay prepared for the 50th anniversary of his own school, Freud (1914:242) remembered his teachers and his experience as a student. He writes:

> We courted them or turned our backs on them, we imagined sympathies and antipathies in them which probably had no existence, we studied their characters and on their's we formed or misinformed our

own. They called up our fiercest opposition and forced us to complete submission; we peered into their little weaknesses, and took pride in their excellences, their knowledge and their justice. At bottom, we felt a great affection for them if they gave us any ground for it, though I cannot tell how many of them were aware of this. But it cannot be denied that our position in regard to them was a quite remarkable one. We were from the very first equally inclined to love and hate them, to criticize and respect them. Psychoanalysis has give the name of "ambivalence" to this readiness to contradictory attitudes, and it has no such difficulty in pointing to the source of ambivalent feelings of such kind.

There is an obvious parallel between the parent and the teacher, the home and the school. This structural similarity suggests a kind of parallel process in which the attitudes and behaviors of both children and adults reflect their previous and current relationships with parents and with their parents' own consciously and unconsciously expressed attitudes towards the school and towards learning.

Psychoanalysis teaches us that memories, like Freud's, come to life in relation to school experience. The expression of memory, in words or behavior, is what Freud called transference. Transference is a way in which people convey—more through behavior than words—a salient quality of experience with their most important primary relationships. Based on our experience of first relationships, our transferences are our unique intrapsychic construction of our interpersonal world. These inner representations of external experience serve as models through which we unwittingly experience most of our future relationships. In other words, transference refers to the complicated ways in which a person perceives others in his current experience as similar in manner to the ways he experienced in past relationships with others. In the transference, the past is never the past but always alive in the present. In this regard, transference refers to the human tendency to organize current experience, usually unwittingly, on the basis of prior experience of past significant relationships.

Michael Basch, a noted psychoanalyst, has reminded us that, "It is the management of the transferences that people have toward us as authorities and/or helpers (and one's reaction to them) that determines how successful both teachers and psychoanalysts will ultimately be in carrying out their respective tasks" (1989:773). The management of the transferences—especially transferences to perceived figures of authority—is complicated by the dynamics of grandiosity, narcissism, ambivalence, persecution and reparation. These dynamics affect the ways in which the different school constituencies perceive themselves and each other. These issues indeed complicate and characterize most relationships among students and teachers, parents and the school, teachers and administrators. Awareness of how these dynamics affect the capacity for forming positive working alliances among these potentially collaborative and conflicting constituencies can mean the difference between hope and despair in the life of a student. The management of these relationships requires schools to develop avenues of approach which do not jeopardize an essential sense of physical and psychological safety. For students, parents and educators to discuss with each other a range of options which are in the best interests of a particular student and/or the school as a whole, all parties need to feel they are working in a reliable and consistent environment of trusted, protective care. In the therapeutic spirit of British pediatrician and psychoanalyst Donald Winnicott, the "good enough school" must find ways to manage the inevitable idealizations, disillusionments, conflicts and efforts to reach reparation which will arise when working with students, parents and teachers.

These transferences tend to be organized around certain psychological themes of interaction and experience: namely, idealization, disillusionment, loss and ambivalence, and reparation. In the next section of our paper, we will provide descriptive examples of the ways these themes are played out in the psychological life of the school.

IDEALIZING THE SCHOOL: THE SCHOOL AS A STAGE FOR DEVELOPMENTAL DRAMAS

The institution of the school is primed to be an object of heightened idealization. Indeed, the very purpose of the school, it has been argued, should be the creation of a world that is better than the "real" world. Writing in 1915, the great philosopher of progressive education, John Dewey, stated that the school must become an ideal place, designed and administered to be a better social environment than the realities of everyday life. Dewey (1916/1966) states:

> . . . it is the business of the school environment to eliminate, so far as possible, the unworthy features of the existing environment from influence upon mental habitudes. It establishes a purified medium of action. Selection aims not only at simplifying but at weeding out what is desirable. Every society gets encumbered with what is trivial, with dead wood from the past, and with what is positively perverse. The school has the duty of omitting such things from the environment which it supplies, and thereby doing what it can to counteract their influence in the ordinary social environment.

The capacity to idealize the other–be it a person or an institution–reflects a never out grown need for a connection with something more powerful than ourselves. Opportunities for idealization and admiration can strengthen an individual's sense of purpose and competence, indeed, allow the person to solidify a coherent sense of self. Successful schools convey an overriding sense of purpose that can help students develop a view of themselves as persons capable of mastering complex materials and situations, making meaningful commitments and engaging in thoughtful action and reflection. The problem with a view of the school as only a "skill development center" is that it disavows the deep emotional connections that make learning truly possible. Learning is often difficult and comes with its fair share of anxiety. When the school stands as an object for idealization, it can allow students, parents, and teachers to stay connected to their work and sustain them through periods of uncertainty and frustration.

Such admiration can also engender feelings of gratitude and generosity. Consider the need schools have for parent volunteers. Parents can participate in a number of vital school functions, especially fund raising. School requests for parent participation are often made on the basis of pragmatic, economic needs for competent no-cost additional labor. Perhaps we do not appreciate fully enough the potential for appealing to parents' own desires for idealization and connection with something that has a larger purpose beyond their own immediate lives. In this regard, we might understand the cynicism teachers and administrators can sometimes feel about parental involvement as a reflection of our own sadness and failure to appreciate ourselves and what we as educators have to offer.

From our perspective the school can and should offer itself to the community of parents, students and teachers as an idealized and idealizable object. One school, for example, has a couple of noteworthy mottos on which it prides itself. One is: "Everything to Help and Nothing to Hinder," a statement which suggests more than a pinch of grandiosity (Frank, 1992a). But aspects of grandiosity can be very beneficial as parents and children need to feel that their educational needs are being addressed in a steady, dependable and even masterful manner. Another motto, inscribed above the stage in the school's auditorium for all to see each day, reads: "A School Should be a Model Home, A Complete Community, An Embryonic Democracy." A clear statement of the school's philosophy, presented in a direct and public manner, allows parents and teachers–but most importantly, students–to reflect on their own experiences in relation to a specific and substantial set of ideals (Frank, 1992b). Such a practice, for example, provides students with a rich tradition of thought and philosophy from which they can begin to think for themselves, making their own interpretations of the legitimacy and fairness of a teacher's actions and/or an administrator's decisions. By providing such ideals, the school not only teaches students the value of high moral standards but also asks, if not expects, students to learn how to question authority in a manner based on sound assessment of the relationship between the ideal and the real.

The identifications established with the school's philosophy not only contribute to the student's growth of character, but also allow parents to solidify a coherent sense of good feeling about themselves as they feel connected to an ideal larger than themselves. In this way, the school can serve as a dependable guiding parental figure to its families. In this transference, old patterns of relating to school persist. For example: Parents want to be good. They want to like teachers and they want to be liked by their children's teachers. They don't want to feel that they have done something wrong and thus may jeopardize the teacher's good feeling toward them. Even highly competent, successful and powerful men and women, can feel anxious and intimidated when a teacher or administrator calls them to talk about a matter concerning their child. They feel as if they themselves had done something wrong; as if they were back in school and were being sent to the principal's office.

Parents display these feelings through an enactment of a variety of transferences. Some parents are extremely compliant, even solicitous. Others can be extremely provocative and challenging in their efforts to show the school and themselves that they are doing the right thing for their children. This tendency is natural, expected and, as we know, psychologically complicated. Behavior can belie questions: Do you like my children? Do you think I am a good parent? Do you like me?

Parents want to feel that they are helping their children and meeting their needs. Parents want to feel that they have done the right thing by having chosen the school as a good enough partner with whom they can share the responsibility of raising and caring for their children. This feeling is heightened especially if parents are paying substantial sums in tuition. Competition for admission to a private school–especially in kindergarten or first grade–can be stiff, and, often with few inner city options available, parents can become desperate to find refuge from large urban public school systems. Almost frantic for shelter, parents are indeed ripe for wishing the school to be great, powerfully competent and unendingly resourceful and caring for their children. In this way, admission to a private school can be experienced by parents as an act of protection and care–aided perhaps by the fortune of good luck and the hand of God.

Freud told us that education, along with government and psychoanalysis, is an impossible profession. And, for these parents, what makes education an impossible profession is the slim chance of having a child admitted to a private school and then being able to pay the ever-rising tuition to keep their child in the school. In this context, parents can also feel that a private school education–almost independent of their child's own academic success–is a sign of self-validation; a sign of their own importance, competence and achievement. Through idealization of the school and/or of themselves, parents develop attachments to the school. Sometimes these attachments convey a greater sense of anxiety and uncertainty than others.

A school can join a parent's idealized fantasies in several ways. The school can–and should–set ideals of high expectations and grandiose claims about what it can accomplish with its students. A school can say that it will do "Everything to Help and Nothing to Hinder"; or that it aims to be "A Model Home, A Complete Community, An Embryonic Democracy." A school can claim it teaches the "whole child," not just a part. It can claim it teaches for more than excellence; it can claim it educates for character. A school can assure parents that it will do more than prepare students for admission to college by teaching students fundamental communication and computational skills. The school can join parents in taking the long view and aim to prepare students for life by working to build self-esteem and develop the courage to take meaningful risks. And schools can aim both to nurture the growth and development of each individual student and develop within each student a deep and lasting sense of care and commitment to the common social good. In short, the school can invite parents and students to participate actively in creating a school environment that is better than the environment of the real world.

Moreover, the school can ask parents to care about their child's education in the same way the school does. It can state that parents should believe in the school's philosophy in the same way that teachers and alumni do. It can claim the moral authority to expect parents to join their children and become involved as active volunteers in the life of the school. The school and the parent each need to feel appreciated by the other. Each needs to see in the face of the other a warm, appreciating, even loving, glow. Parents want to feel they are being good parents; teachers want to feel they are doing a good job. For a variety of reasons, each party can feel uneasy and doubtful about their own competence in the roles they assume. Pointing to the state of our nation's public schools and to the growing numbers of children who grow up poor in our country, many educators believe that children are not especially valued in our culture. Accordingly, they argue, adults who work with children are not afforded much meaningful social status. Consequently, teachers can feel uneasy and vulnerable about their own self-esteem when working with wealthy, powerful parents, who in their own right, can have their own grandiose notions about themselves and their children's capabilities.

Private schools are removed, for the most part, from the desperation and futility felt by so many whose lives are affected by life in inner city public schools. Yet, even in our more exclusive and less chaotic schools, children and families can experience their own social and psychological troubles which affect the ways in which parents and schools struggle to develop positive working relationships. Even in these schools, that promote a public presentation of warm, family-like relationships, different personal histories and different roles tend to promote different world views and competing interpretations about what parents and the school need to do in order to be helpful to the children of our schools. In schools, as in all societies, cooperation and competition are both intregral aspects of human relationships. And yet, it is especially difficult in schools that pride themselves on good will, cooperative spirit and a shared sense of democratic citizenship to recognize and acknowledge the presence of hostile and aggressive feelings toward fellow community members: students, parents, colleagues. Schools and parents are logical and essential partners in the lives of children. As in any relationship, however, the parent-school relationship is vulnerable to irrational responses shaped by the transferences each party brings to their encounters with others.

Yet, as long as parents feel the school is living up to their own wished for perceptions of the school as a place where promises are kept and needs are cared for, the school will continue to be idealized. And as long as the school feels parents appreciate its efforts to care for and educate their children, the school can maintain itself as an idealizable figure in the lives of families.

Things are fine as long as things are fine.

But what happens when something goes wrong? What happens to the student-parent-school relationship when a child develops problems and is having difficulty thriving in the school? Or what happens when, in a normative manner, a student enters his adolescence at the same time as his parents begin to see the world through middle-aged eyes? Whether the school's inquiry is about a student's own struggles to excel or a parent's difficulty in giving their child the space needed for growth to occur, it is important to consider how any action or communication might affect the psychological balance of adult narcissism and self-esteem.

As a symbol, the school evokes powerful feelings among children and adults. The idea of the school calls forth ideals of promise, purity and hope, a world free from contaminations that plague everyday social life. Yet the reality of the school–no matter how good a school–can not at all times and in all cases live up to its stated or attributed ideal. Mythology must give way to the inevitability of disillusionment.

DISILLUSIONMENT, LOSS AND AMBIVALENCE

Schooling is an emotionally charged business. Perhaps more than any other enterprise, schools are charged with the care of parents' often most cherished and precious connection to life: their children as representations of themselves; as representations of their own unique sense of self. In this context, children are not their own persons. A student in a classroom is not simply a student in a chair, at a desk, taking notes, passing notes or staring out the window. That young person exists, in some form, as an extension of all that has gone right and all that has gone wrong in his or her parents' lives. A student's school experience can represent parental anxieties about success and failure as well as generations of family hopes and dreams for a better future. And that is not all. A student in a classroom is also likely to serve as a reflection of the teacher's own sense of competence as a professional and as a person. Independent of each individual parent and teacher's own unique personality, there exists a normative psychological climate in which students, parents, teachers and administrators are likely to experience each other as persons who either help or hinder the maintenance of his or her own self-esteem.

Children can make parents feel acutely vulnerable. When the school begins to question a child's functioning, parents can easily take matters painfully to heart. Inquiry into our children's actions can make us feel anxious and ambivalent. In these inquiries, we tell stories and make interpretations. Our accounts portray our desire to challenge and respond as well as our fear of risk and the unknown. Our constructions demonstrate our ability to retain balance and lose our footing. In our statements, and in what we hear of other people's statements, we struggle with the tendency to reveal and to conceal. What we ask and what we question betray our wish to know and our wish not to know. In the same single moment, we can seek knowledge and understanding and we can tenaciously subvert that very search.

For example, parents can appreciate the school's interest and attention given to their child. Yet, parents also experience–in a heightened and exaggerated way–the school's inquiry as a criticism of their ability to raise children. And they can experience a call from a teacher, dean, counselor or principal as a rejection, as an abandonment by the school of its relationship to the family as a caring parental figure. In this regard, questions are perceived as an attack; inquiry as a form of persecution. In their anguish and distress, it becomes difficult, if only for a period of time, for parents to tolerate and manage ambivalent feelings; to balance their feelings of love and hate, appreciation and rage at the school.

These issues are heightened even more when the school is in the process of considering whether or not it will counsel a student out of the school. Despite–and perhaps because of–seemingly strong prior attachments to the school, talk of counseling out is almost always experienced by parents as a disruptive life event which leaves them feeling suddenly and unexpectedly traumatized and humiliated. Despite significant and methodical assessment, if the school feels it can no longer meet the child's developmental needs–and that it is in the best interest of the child to attend a different school–parents can nonetheless feel that the school is not living up to its claim of: "Everything to help and nothing to hinder." They feel they have been cruelly assaulted and heartlessly abandoned. They feel they have been ruthlessly betrayed.

School personnel, on the other hand, are likely to perceive their own actions on behalf of the school as consistent with the school's educational philosophy. Even as staff might have to manage potential feelings of ambivalence and guilt, the school would need to proceed with its decision that to hold on to a student whose needs it can no longer meet would be irresponsible and hindering to the child's development. From this perspective, to counsel a student out would represent every effort on the part of the school to help parents understand the need to find an alternative educational setting which can more appropriately meet their child's needs.

Clearly, not all parents experience the school's inquiry as an attack. In many cases, parents are relieved to hear from the school. Parents may have had their own concerns about one of their children and may have felt additional anxiety when interpreting the school's silence as a sign of the school's lack of empathic awareness; that the school was neither observant nor concerned enough about their child. As one parent said, "I'm so glad you called. We've been terribly worried. We just thought the school didn't care."

The school, at times, is no less vulnerable to feeling attacked by the presence of a question. "What is going on in that math class?" "Why did that teacher speak to my child that way?" "What kind of 'model home' is this place?" "Who is in charge here, anyway?" "You know, until this thing happened with my daughter, I loved this school, I was really in love with this school. But now, I just don't know. I'm really afraid that I am falling out of love." Parental disillusionment about a teacher's functioning or about an administrative decision has the potential to make school staff feel angry, vulnerable and attacked, hurt and unappreciated. There is, in schools, a strong sense shared by staff, that *we* are the professionals, the educators; that the curriculum is *our* domain. *We* are the authorities: "Don't ask us questions, don't tell us what to do," and, as the old line goes, "Just drop your kid off the day after Labor Day and pick him up around the beginning of June." When pride and self-esteem are injured, powerful and ambivalent feelings can arise. School people want extensive autonomy but they also can feel enraged when they think parents are not doing their job and instead are turning to the school to take on even more roles that were once reserved for the family, the physician or the church. In schools where parents are encouraged to participate in the life of the school, this contrary and ambivalent attitude poses some very real conflicts.

The roots of human ambivalence can be found in the early experience of our first relationships. One should not, therefore, be surprised to find that the anxiety of inquiry permeates the earliest moments in the school's relationship with a family. It can become no small concern to the school to know whether a family has sent their child to the school because of the parents' deep belief and allegiance to the school's philosophy or because the school was one of the very few alternatives to big city public education. A marriage of convenience, not a union of love. Their narcissism injured, their sense of specialness rejected, persons in the school can feel devalued, unappreciated, victimized. Unable to acknowledge their own rage at parents, school staff can project an image of parents as a hostile, unreasonable group, ready to take siege of the school, fire its faculty, change its philosophy, rewrite its very history, even give the school a new name.

These feelings represent fantasies organized around a social defense (Hirschhorn, 1988) where anxiety is contained by separating good from bad feelings and attributing one's own unacknowledged negative feelings to another group. This emotional configuration can inform the school's sometimes unwitting tendency to imagine parents as feeling hostile in routine evening parent meetings, individual parent conferences and, of course, in certain phone calls with parents.

Recently, in one school, a series of brightly colored, well-designed posters appeared in the halls and other public places in the school. Printed in bold and appealing graphics, each of the nearly forty signs contained a different appealing black and white photograph of students and teachers engaged in learning and playing, and a different quotation culled from various students, teachers and parents associated with the school over its ninety year history. These quotations contributed to the dynamic feeling of life in the halls. In a visually appealing way, the posters added an important historical dimension to the fast pace of contemporary school life. The posters gave us a sense that the work of today is connected to ideals of the past. The project was conceived and designed by parents and staff associated with the school's Development Office. The idea for the project stemmed directly from the concern that too many current parents do not adequately understand the nature and mission of the school. The aim was to help promote a more effective way to educate parents about the values and philosophy of the school. But more to the point, the project's purpose was to respond to the school's feeling that its philosophy, its curriculum and its personnel—were not truly appreciated. Freud taught us how appearance disguises other dimensions of reality: the happy colors and lofty ideals posted around the school were efforts to transform the darker feelings of injury, abandonment and powerlessness.

For these very reasons of vulnerable self-regard, and its manifested defenses, school staff can fall prey to avoiding calling a family when a student is experiencing marked difficulty. To call is to add one more case to one's busy and often overloaded schedule. To call is to come to terms with a full range of conflicting feelings about what it means to be caretaker. To call is to admit one's limitations; that one has failed in an heroic act and cannot care for the child alone. To call is to face the anxieties of letting go; of facing more directly possible lurking feelings of hostility and aggression toward the child, the family, and perhaps even colleagues in the school. To call is to acknowledge an elation of relief at having finally disposed of a long-term problem; and to call is to feel the guilt of failure and the humiliation of having to ask for help from an unconsciously perceived enemy. Who says schools aren't a part of the real world?

Yet every good teacher knows parental ambivalence governs the relationship to the school and the responses to the children as students. Each parent, like each teacher, approaches school with a romantic structure seemingly filled with hope and optimism, only in time to give way to some measure of disillusionment. It is interesting to note in this regard how often one can hear parents rationalize policies like letter grades for elementary school students with reference to the "real world," as if childhood were somehow divorced from reality. One would imagine that most children would find such an idea surprising. This suggests the degree to which adults are alienated from their own experience of childhood and, for our purposes, from the emotional significance of the school itself, from the very disillusionment some parents seem to feel they need to introduce in the name of "reality." In one way or another, the tendency to have our children repeat our own experience is a powerful one. It is precisely this repetition and alienation that psychoanalysis seeks to understand. How parents experience that disillusionment and how that disillusionment is experienced by students and teachers is very much of interest to the school that must contain and modulate its effects and its expression.

Adapting to change can be a difficult matter. Periods of transition can make people feel anxious about the loss and growth they may be feeling (Marris, 1974/1979). Change is structured into the life of even the most conservative schools, making students, teachers and parents experience feelings of separation at those moments marked by transition in grade level or other developmental milestones. How a school manages transitions within its organizational structure can affect the degree to which members of the school community can feel anxious and disillusioned. Parents, for example, often experience the transitions from lower school to middle school and from middle school to high school in a traumatic manner. In a JK through 12 school, parents of kindergarten and lower school children tend to experience the school as a warm and welcoming place. The transition to middle school is often experienced by parents in a manner which makes them feel suddenly thwarted, even assaulted. Parents can react to such changes as middle school students receiving letter grades for the first time; fewer formally scheduled parent-teacher conferences than in lower school; and teacher's written evaluative comments tend to be shorter and less detailed than the comments written by lower school teachers. Parents can feel they have less of a textured understanding of what their children are doing than they had in lower school. They can feel they are being left out.

The transition to high school can be experienced in a similar manner. Teachers in the upper grades can be resentful of parental involvement, feeling that older students need to learn to take responsibility for their own learning. In this message, teacher and student communicate to parents a desire for the young adolescent to develop a significant relationship outside of the home. Parents can experience this kind of high school message as insensitive to parental needs to maintain a sense of control and supervision over their child's life. And, understandably, it is not easy for parents to find comfortable ways to let go.

Each school has an ethos, and each school's ethos is reflected in the emotional tone or structure of the school. Such an emotional structure embodies a complex and highly condensed expression of the school's collective experience. This experience is influenced both by the wide variety of idiosyncratic interpretations of the school held by members of the school community and by the normative developmental shifts students, teachers and parents experience as students move from childhood to adolescence and as adults enter middle-age and beyond.

Each school, therefore, needs to look at its policies and how those policies or practices might affect the manner in which its constituencies experience those changes and transitions which are structured into the life of the school. Yet just as the students must contend with their feelings of loss as they experience the inevitable changes school life can bring, so must their parents and teachers struggle to understand how they feel about change in school.

ROMANCE AND RITUAL IN THE SENIOR YEAR

In schools, no year is perhaps fraught with the potential for dramatic ambivalence of feeling than the senior year of high school (Thompson, 1990). For most parents and students, the senior year marks the time when the end of childhood becomes palpable. The year is defined by a range of developmental transitions in which students and parents feel joy and sadness which comes with growth, loss and separation. Let us recall Freud's words about child and adolescent development: "The freeing of an individual, as he grows up, from the authority of his parents is one of the most necessary though one of the most painful results brought about by the course of development." The cumulative effect of this year on the lives of twelfth grade teachers and administrators should also not be underestimated.

During this year, students, teachers and parents traverse the terrain of many feelings. They are each prone to idealize aspects of themselves and others. They also can feel the pain of disillusionment and seek restitution of hurt feelings and damaged relationships, all in an effort to try to hold all these many feelings together in some liveable and meaningfully integrated manner. The senior year, like any stage of school experience, is shaped by experiences of separation and relationship; and each school experience is the stage on which the drama of separation and relation is played. School traditions, interestingly, can provide us with just such a stage. Understanding what is communicated by those who participate in the ritual of a school tradition can bring telling insights into the psychological dynamics which exist in a school's culture. Such traditions—the events we almost blindly take for granted and reenact each year with each new group of students—can present themselves like fragments from a dream open for interpretation and understanding (Stein, 1994; Gabriel, 1994).

At one school, seniors engage in several longstanding school traditions. These traditions are used by each new group of seniors as opportunities to express unconscious feelings about their relationship to themselves and others. Each tradition, like a single dream fragment, can be analyzed for its unique manifest and latent content. Yet, a series of traditions, or rituals, like a string of dream fragments, can be read together as if they comprised a more unified and coherent expression of anxiety and desire.

The senior year begins with anxiety and romance. Seniors typically approach the end of their junior year and beginning of their senior year with outward feelings of hopeful and uneasy anticipation, if not excitement. Many see their senior year as the culminating moment of their secondary school experience. Many see it as a time to realize goals. Others are a bit more desperate to make up for mishaps of the past. Nearly all are preoccupied, even if in denial, about setting a course for the next few years. Yet as the oldest students in the school, many students also harbor feelings which are a mixture of aggression and delight. The senior year is their time to have long-awaited access to key roles in school traditions, traditions reserved for seniors. At last, first choice preferences and high status will go to them. Finally, they can lay claim to the privileged access of seniority and power. With the desire of entitlement and the might of firstborn birthrights, they feel that they have finally made it. Many state that they believe their senior year will be the best year of their lives.

The romance has begun. From the start, students idealize the year, and consequently, aspects of themselves. And the school joins them. For example, at one school, the first major school tradition of the year highlights seniors in the second week of school. The tradition, called "Big Brothers and Sisters," involves the seniors selecting a lower or middle school class to which each senior can become a "big brother" or "big sister." With an unwitting sense of foreshadowing, on the stage of the school's auditorium, the school organizes an all-school assembly in which seniors sit on the stage in the same raised-tier format they will use at their graduation in June. At this assembly, the school community learns which seniors have selected to be big brothers or sisters to which middle or lower school classes. The school community also hears how the seniors have chosen to introduce and describe each twelfth grader to their new little brothers and sisters and to others in the audience. The seniors tell mysterious, inside jokes and use private nicknames known only to a handful of fellow seniors. Younger students both marvel at these mysterious communications and idealize the seniors because of the mystery they have constructed. Younger students and other members of the audience also feel separated from the seniors because they do not understand–nor were they meant to fully understand–the inside jokes and nicknames. The seniors' manner of presenting themselves speaks to their own sense of ambivalence. They aim to connect with the audience, allowing the younger students to idealize them. And they aim to separate themselves from the audience, allowing their anxieties about their impending departure to serve as a communication to the school regarding their current feelings of isolation, disconnection and confusion.

Although the tradition is aimed mostly to benefit the younger students, the event of the announcement is designed as a time to honor and recognize the seniors. This event also represents a foreshadowing of things to come. As seniors begin further preparation for college visits and writing college applications, this ritual event is a preview of powerful wishes for public admiration, acceptance and recognition; a validation from the external world of their intrinsic value and worth.

The day of the big brothers and sisters ceremony begins with a special breakfast for seniors. Kindergarten students arrive at the breakfast held in the senior class' homeroom to distribute to twelfth graders colored t-shirts the school has purchased for each of them. During the preceding week, a faculty committee has coordinated an effort throughout the lower school to produce bright and colorful art which a group of teachers uses to decorate and display in the senior class' homeroom and in the school's auditorium, the site of the celebration. The ceremony begins when the seniors, dressed in their t-shirts, enter a darkened, standing-room-only school auditorium audience lead by the beam of a spotlight and the thunder of two bag pipers playing. The crowd, now on its feet, cheers and claps for the seniors as they parade through the aisles and toward their seats on stage. It doesn't get much better than this.

As a class, the seniors next return to the stage three weeks later. At that time, the entire school gathers in the school's auditorium in preparation for the next major school tradition, a fall festival called "County Fair." County Fair is fun-loving enterprise, run largely by students, where students and parents can shop at booths sponsored by each grade level, listen to live music, watch a student-directed play, and more. Ideals mark the day. Students are very aware, committed and proud, that the proceeds from the Fair go to support the school's financial aid-scholarship fund.

The school then picks up where it left off. Two days before County Fair, each grade level performs a brief skit on the stage of the school's auditorium to an audience of the entire school. The aim of the skits is for each grade level to do a bit of advertizing to inform the rest of the school community of the product it is selling, the service it is offering or the activity it is sponsoring. The spirit of personal involvement, group solidarity and community idealization is high. The County Fair skits begin with the presence of the youngest students, the 4 year old junior kindergartners.

They are cute and charming. As they take their place on stage, endearing sighs of "ahhhh" come from their older school mates. Sibling relationships seem sound. The presentation of skits proceeds in order of chronological age, the seniors coming last. However, as the 10th and then the 11th graders present their skits, the audience's mood begins to change. Something significant is about to shift. In the 11th grade skit, a rivalry emerges between the 11th and 12th graders. In their skit, the 11th graders advertize that the food they will be selling at County Fair is better than the food the seniors will be selling, thus making the juniors a better, morally superior group of persons. The seniors, of course, claim that their product is better and that the seniors themselves are indeed superior. And since they are the oldest, their skit is performed last, giving seniors the final, ultimate word. Worried that they might be rejected in the large pond of college applicants and beyond, seniors seek reassurance of their competencies by asserting their strength in the smaller, familiar pool of their own school. In this way, hostility and aggression replace the cute and charming. In the face of fearing that they will be crushed by the "real world," the seniors take a preemptive strike to assert their authority and strength in the "better world" of the school. Fearing aggression from outside, they identify with the threat they perceive and lay claim to all that comes in their path. In the skit the seniors perform, the psychological stance of the school in relation to its 12th graders moves unconsciously from idealization to disillusionment.

The skit occurs on the eve of a long fall weekend when most seniors travel to visit colleges. The senior class' skit is a truly fascinating unconscious enactment of their collective anxieties. In their skit, they unwittingly revive the worries that have been lying at the edge of awareness: the impending separation from home and school. This is a fear perhaps felt especially intensely by those students who have been at the school for fourteen years, since the time when they were once the cute and charming junior kindergartners. Without being aware of the content of what they are presenting, seniors enact in their skit scenes demonstrating regressive, counter-phobic responses to their anxieties as well as unwitting expression of their own sense of loss and disillusionment about the fantasied promise of the year.

Each year, the seniors stage a skit which the faculty find intensely offensive, crude, and inappropriate for a school audience. During the Fair, seniors run a food stand where the featured item on the menu is the hot dog. The general motif of the seniors' lengthy skit about the hot dogs they are going to sell includes explicit dramatizations of a range of oral and phallic themes: sexual exploitation, aggression, domination, narcissism, regression, each one highlighted by improvisations of their own immaturity (Frank, 1990). While students seem open to the manifest messages these competing skits communicate, faculty members experience these skits, especially the seniors' skit, as a sudden, shocking betrayal of profound trusts. Teachers expect seniors to act responsibly; after all, they argue, that was the implicit significance of the ritual "big brothers and sisters" ceremony. The free space of student organized activities–activities which claim no direct guidance or supervision by teachers or administrators–can be perceived or experienced by adults as running counter to their constant efforts to encourage, if not insist, that students be well mannered in public, respectful and concerned about the lives of others beyond their own immediate circle of relationships.

Yet, for adults, the provocative content and style of the skits, can, as well, resonate with current developmental issues of loss, control and sexuality in their own lives. The skits can evoke in adults feelings of envy, shame and guilt over their own unconscious reactions to the aggressive and sexual content presented in the skits. Faculty complaints of outrage or boredom in regard to the skit can suggest an emotional distancing from the aggressive, sexual and narcissistic nature of the senior skits. Such feelings can include the unanalyzed world of adult sexual and aggressive fantasies about their adolescent students. The anger and disregard for the meaning of these skits–which eventually lead high school teachers to intervene and alter the way in which the seniors perform their skits–suggest adult anxiety about perceived threats to their authority, their self-esteem and their mortality. Each senior class, after all, can serve as an uncomfortable reminder to teachers and administrators that they are not getting any younger. And, once again, schools that pride themselves on developing cooperative, model citizens have trouble understanding or accepting public expression of conflict, competition, aggressive hostility, anxious insecurity and counter-phobic regression.

Faculty response also indicates a fall from the grace of positive idealizations which had characterized their perceptions of the seniors when they were on stage only a couple of weeks earlier. Each year the seniors have, unwittingly, enacted this fantasy; and each year the faculty has decried the seniors and voiced their profound disappointment in them. The disillusionment has become ritualized, indeed, institutionalized. The seniors seek ways to express their uncertainties about growing up and the school holds fast to its idealized view of itself and its expectations for the seniors which the school had ritualized only a few weeks earlier when seniors were given the responsibility to act as mature role models for the younger students. Each year the wish appears. Each year the wish goes unfulfilled. The school enacts the repetition once again, as if setting itself up for disappointment. Perhaps it is less painful to let go if one feels that the person departing isn't so great, after all. Spoiling sets the stage for separation.

Sure enough, though, the school, also unwittingly, tries it once again a few months later. The pain of disillusionment gives way for the return of the wish to idealize. On the morning of the day the school breaks for Christmas vacation, the school calls on the seniors to come before the school community to perform another school ritual. The senior class puts on its annual presentation of "The Twelve Days of Christmas." There is pageantry, elegance, humor, tenderness, slapstick comedy, demonstrations of feminine flirtation and masculine prowess. Lower school children perform songs they have been preparing. A senior dressed as Santa Claus thrills the audience with his ritualized surprise entrance. In this ritual, the seniors are on stage, in the limelight, and loving it. And so is their audience. Parents, knowing that this might be their last chance to see their senior child perform, have cameras and video recorders in hand.

All this occurs only hours before a two week vacation is to begin. Spirits around the school are quite high. Yet, on the eve of separation, the darker side of parting also presents itself. At the brink of separation, the school wishes to idealize the seniors as a way to rehearse for the eventual departure and loss which will happen at graduation in June. In this way, idealization can be understood as a way to cope with the pain of anxiety and the sadness of loss. The seniors, of course, are still, understandably in flux and feeling uncertain about their futures. By mid-December, a few seniors have been accepted to college. Most, however, have only begun to complete and mail their applications. At just that moment when the school calls on them to act as responsible role models for the rest of the school, and become symbolic representations of the schools highest ideals as reflected in their performance in "The Twelve Days of Christmas," seniors continue to feel ambivalent about moving ahead. What goes unspoken among the crowd of students, teachers and parents is the fact that most seniors are performing without having slept the night before. After rehearsing late into the evening, the entire senior class gathers at the home of a classmate where, with at least some parental supervision, they stay up all night, supposedly to make the traditional popcorn balls for their little brothers and sisters in the lower and middle school, as the seniors themselves also engage in and perpetuate a long standing, self-made ritual of all night drinking and partying.

"The Twelve Days of Christmas," hallowed tradition in the school, symbol of senior status and opportunity to shine before the ideals of the school, is also an expression of the pervading ambivalence and disillusionment seniors feel about themselves and the significant changes which lie before them. And, in its own way, so does the school. From the Big Brother and Sister ceremony to the Senior Skit to "The Twelve Days of Christmas," the school, unwittingly, enacts the drama of separation and loss for all to see and experience. Each moment represents efforts to come to terms with the parting of the senior class, and with each class, so, too, leaves a part of each teacher who has taught this group of students.

Seniors next gather together as a group for an event called "The Senior Adulation Dinner." This dinner was originally conceived by senior parents and students as an event to honor those who have taught the seniors over the years. It was conceived as a time for the seniors to express their gratitude and thanks–to adulate–their teachers from kindergarten through high school. In the first few years of this tradition, senior parents spent long hours decorating the school's lunchroom, transforming it into a lovely space for a formal dinner and student testimonials expressing appreciation to their teachers.

In time, however, a shift occurred, perhaps in keeping with the greed and narcissism of the 1980s. For a number of years, the dinner was moved off of the common ground of the school to the glamour of fancy downtown restaurants. There, the "Senior Adulation Dinner" became an event to which teachers were invited, but the focus of honor was moved from teachers to the seniors themselves. More recent senior classes have shifted back once again, bringing the event back to the school and the focus back to the teachers, offering seniors, parents and teachers a ritualized forum for seeking restitution and reparation of feelings toward themselves and others.

Yet, interestingly, even as the event has regained its original intent, where seniors and parents aim to express genuine feelings of appreciation and where healing hopes to overcome ambivalence, residue of a darker side perhaps remains. Webster's Dictionary tells us that "adulate" means "to praise too highly or flatter servilely" and that "servile" means "like or characteristic of a slave; humbly yielding or submissive; suggesting the cringing, submissive behavior characteristic of a slave."

Implicit in the concept of adulation is the concept of power and authority in human relationships. Our feelings about power can be complicated, ambivalent and contradictory. Someone has more power than someone else. Someone wishes one had more power and control than someone else. Someone wishes for the other to have more power than oneself. Whether power is perceived in one's own hands or in the hands of another, the presence or absence of power can evoke feelings of persecution and/or protection.

On the eve of their graduation, perhaps in addition to wanting to make peace with their real and fantasied teachers, seniors may be expressing a wish for adults to remain in control, to reassert their prior roles as authority figures in their lives as the anxiety of freedom and more independence may be especially frightening. Seniors may also be expressing a simultaneous and difficult to acknowledge desire for increased autonomy and that that wish still has traces of aggressive overtones where the wish itself expresses loving and hateful feelings toward perceived or once perceived powerful adults. In this wish, where autonomy is still laced with feelings of aggression, seniors desire to rid themselves from the control and power of adults and instead wish for a change in roles where the seniors become the dominators and the teachers become the dominated.

In their effort to separate from home and school, seniors struggle to separate themselves from structures of power which includes the structure of power itself. Perhaps without a full sense of awareness, seniors are seeking a way to relate to themselves and others which might free them from the structures of much of their prior perceived experience where human relationships have been defined by either having almost magical control over their lives or being utterly subservient to the mercy of powerful and hostile adult figures. Somewhere between all or nothing lies the potential for a more integrated stance in relation to others.

Each of these ritualized school traditions–Big Brothers and Sisters, the County Fair Skits, "The Twelve Days of Christmas," the Senior Adulation Dinner–are emblematic acts which represent part of the process by which the school tries to integrate its perceptions and feelings about the senior class, in particular, and human relationships, in general. And, in the final weeks of school, the seniors, once again, engage in collective regressive behavior in two more senior rituals–Senior Ditch Day (seniors cut classes) and the Senior Prank (where seniors create and execute a large and secret practical joke on the school). Yet, by the time of graduation in June, seniors can begin to appreciate their new status and separate from the school. The school staff can come to appreciate and understand the seniors' expression of maturity and immaturity. In this sense, for the adults in the school, graduation stands for the reparation and integration of positive and negative feelings about seniors and themselves.

The senior year can also be marked by tensions between parents and the school. Conflicts can arise over the college admissions process, the courses a student takes and the grades a senior receives. At an unconscious level, parents may feel that the school has taken their child away from them and hold the school responsible for the sadness that such separation brings. In addition, parents, struggling with their own midlife developmental issues, can feel disappointed if their children do not fulfill specific goals and wishes that they themselves would like to have realized in their own lives. In this context, school personnel must be prepared to absorb the anger, disappointment and sadness of parents and students, as well as their own feelings of loss and appreciation for their students and for themselves as teachers.

THE EMOTIONAL STRUCTURE OF THE SCHOOL: TOWARDS A REPARATIVE PROCESS

The examples illustrate salient dynamics of the senior year and how *the school romance* offers us a way to understand the powerful emotional ambivalence that characterizes our experience of school. The rapid shifts from responsibility to regression, from idealization to disillusionment, from denial to recognition reflect a complex, never fully resolved emotional constellation involving our efforts to manage the pain and sorrow of loss and the inevitability of change. How can the school assist students, teachers and parents in this process?

Reparation is a strong force in human experience (Klein, 1936/64). Just as guilt over feelings of envy, frustration and anger is inevitable so is a reparative process that reflects a desire for integration and healing. The demands of academic achievement and the challenges of social life result in such painful feelings often expressed in the child's and adult's relation to the school. We find ourselves feeling angry because we were not recognized as we felt we should be and feel envy towards those who are rewarded. These feelings are the natural consequence of social life. To try to control expressions of such frustration completely can only lead to a repressive atmosphere and a necessary denial of our own inner experience.

Failure to respond to hostile and destructive behavior, however, robs us of the opportunity to experience guilt and to transform that experience into reparative activity. Constructive involvements and doing for others allow us to reclaim feelings of love and generosity both for ourselves and towards those who have excited our envy and anger. We all know how life is complicated by its contradictions, how we can love and hate the same person at the same time. We know how it feels to be frazzled, overwhelmed and feeling divided; how it feels to live with ambivalence; and how that tension is part of what it means to be human. As individuals, each of us strives to balance the many different responsibilities and feelings we have. In this way, we are each trying to integrate better our own personal lives. In a world so often marked by uncertainty, disorder and disintegration, each of us nonetheless struggles to feel coherent, organized, whole. When we are able to acknowledge those painful feelings which we have split-off and projected on to others, and instead retain those feelings in a more integrated and balanced manner, we have the opportunity to be better situated psychologically to understand another person's experience in a caring and empathic manner. The school must try to find a way not only to provide understanding but also to establish a structure in which students, parents and teachers can express, in an integrated manner, their loving and generous impulses.

The emotional significance of the school in our lives can help us recognize the ambivalence that often influences the day-to-day experience of school. In the senior year example, the structure of the school plays a crucial role in facilitating and giving recognition to the complex emotions that make an event like graduation so powerful. Here we see the value of ritual and tradition in relation to the reparative process. Ritual provides a constant and anticipated structure for the expression of anticipation and disappointment, joy and sadness. The school has a clear role in providing and maintaining such structures. Of course, these very traditions and rituals are subject to the very ambivalence they are designed to contain.

The school must serve to contain *the school romance* so that it can be expressed in ways that keep alive the meanings of the school and our efforts to come to terms with ourselves as students, educators, and as people. The school must be prepared to absorb the great expectations, sadness and disappointment of students, parents and colleagues. It is in this sense that the school must provide what Donald Winnicott describes as "the good enough holding environment." "Good enough" does not mean adequate or average quality of education. The "good enough" school strives for excellence and improvement. The "good enough" school has depth, substance and solidity to provide students, teachers and parents with informed guidance and leadership through both the expected and unexpected elements of disorder, uncertainty and conflict that come with everyday school life. The school cannot resolve all conflicts or satisfy all longings. The school cannot change itself to meet the latest demand for one thing or another. Since we wish so much from the school, since *the school romance* excites such powerful desire and feelings of ambivalence within ourselves, our students, our children and for our school itself, the school must struggle to stand firm. Hopefully, in some measure, a kind of recognition can be achieved. As the poet Wallace Stevens reminds us, "Imperfection is our paradise."

Ritual provides an opportunity for a kind of reparative process to take place. While disappointment can give rise to envy and hatred, so, too, can the acceptance of such feelings lead to the desire to want to restore and repair. Nothing is more corrosive than to have to live with feelings of anger and envy and to be without opportunities to act in ways that allow for the expression of love and gratitude. Without such opportunities, cynicism develops. The school can play an important role in helping students, parents and teachers to experience a greater sense of integration as individuals–and as a community–through various kinds of collaborative efforts that draw upon powerful feelings of admiration and gratitude. We all want to be able to give of ourselves and, by so doing, feel that the world is a better place.

The everyday experience of school life includes a complex social arena of developmental, age, racial, ethnic, class, gender and cohort differences influenced by each school's own set of routine social practices, rituals and traditions. These issues, however, represent more than current social categories. They represent powerful expectations, assumptions imbued with desire, world views full of affect and emotional complications resonating with prior experiences at home and in school. The reactions students, teachers and parents have to these issues, and to their own and others' emotional residue, inform how they feel about authority figures, the school and the role of schooling in our society.

Understanding the psychodynamics of *the school romance* can help educators recognize and interpret the variety of meanings that rise from the personal, developmental and social issues that can be at play in the school setting. This perspective should not obscure or rationalize the actual problems that social life brings. Rather, an appreciation of *the school romance* can help us conceptualize the inevitable, normal responses to the experience of the school and, therefore, help us to develop a tolerance and empathy for these most human of responses. Understanding the dynamic nature of how individuals and groups make sense of their respective experiences in schools can contribute to the creation and the maintenance of a school community that is responsive and understanding in its relations with students, parents and teachers.

We need also to remember that beyond our own private memories, associations and responses to school life lie the more public–yet no less powerful–evocations of the school expressed by adults in economic, social and ideological terms. Our personal experience of the school is also informed by the values and conflicts that comprise the broader culture in which we live. Americans have long had high hopes for the role of education in our society. The school has been idealized as a place of potential and possibility, an institution that can provide real opportunities that can improve the quality of life. Indeed, as historian David Cohen (1976) notes, the very history of the American school is shaped by projected wishes for the school to heal the experienced trauma of modern life. Through the institution of the school, parents and policymakers have sought reparation from that which they feel we as a society have lost first to industrialization and urbanization and now to the disillusionment of America's global prowess, the decay of our domestic social and economic institutions, and the deepening retrenchment of the underclass. In a world where many feel they have little control over their lives, Americans, nonetheless, persevere in their capacities to cope with these and other social changes. In the hope of building a better way of life, we still need to believe in the promise of education and the idea that the school can be a symbol of recovery, an object to which we continue to attach our wish to recapture the supportive bond of community, real or imagined, that we continue to envision, idealize and mourn.

NOTES

1. Our thinking about the subjective experience of school life is informed by understandings of human relationships developed in the clinical situation of psychoanalysis. Psychoanalysis is both a method of inquiry and a body of theory about individual and group experience that is able to help us interpret the meaning of life stories and understand something of the complexities of human experience throughout the life course. Psychoanalytically informed understandings about human relationships can offer us avenues of approach to illuminate the deeply subjective nature of learning and the psychological significance of the relationships that structure school life. These relationships include those among teacher and student, parent and school, teacher and administrator. More specifically, psychoanalysis offers us a method and a theory for understanding how the past lives on in our present attitudes toward the institution of the school–and toward the experience of learning in general–and in the meanings which the teacher and the school continue to have for us as adults.

2. *A Special Relationship: Our Teachers and How We Learned.* (1991) Board: Pushcart Press, 17-18.

REFERENCES

Basch, Michael Franz (1989). The teacher, the transference and development. In *Learning and Education: Psychoanalytic Perspectives.* Madison: International Universities Press. 1989. eds. Field, Kay, Cohler, Bertram and Wool, Glorye.

Cohen, David K. (1976). Loss as a theme in social policy. Harvard Educational Review: Vol. 46, No. 4. November.

Dewey, John (1916/1966). *Democracy and Education*. New York: The Free Press.

Frank, Daniel B. (1990). Unpublished. Improvisations of the immature: Ritual, regression and adolescent development in a school tradition. Francis W. Parker School.

—— (1992a). Everything to help, nothing to hinder: Grandiosity, ambivalence and boundaries in the parent-school alliance. *Residential Treatment for Children & Youth.*

—— (1992b). Unpublished. How schools can help children of divorce: Psychoanalytic perspectives on school experience.

Freud, Sigmund (1908). Family romances. Standard Edition. Volume 9. London: Hogarth Press, 1959, pp. 237-241.

—— (1914). Some reflections on schoolboy psychology. Standard Edition. Volume 13. London: Hogarth Press. 1955. pp. 241-244.

Fuqua, Paula B. (1993). A model of the learning process based on self psychology. In *Emotions and Learning Reconsidered: International Perspectives*. Eds. Field, Kay, Kaufman, Edward and Saltzman, Charles. New York: Gardner Press.

Gabriel, Yiannis (1994). The organizational dreamworld: Workplace stories, fantasies and subjectivity. In *Psychoanalytic Interpretations of Organizational Cultures*. Papers published by the International Society for the Psychoanalytic Study of Organizations.

Hirschhorn, Larry (1988). *The Workplace Within: Psychodynamics of Organizational Life*. Cambridge: MIT Press.

Klein, Melanie (1936/1964). Love, guilt and reparation. In *Love, Hate and Reparation*. New York: Norton.

Salzberger-Wittenberg, Isca, Henry, Gianna and Osborne, Elsie (1983). *The Emotional Experience of Learning and Teaching*. London: Routledge.

Stein, Howard (1994). Workplace organizations and culture theory: A psychoanalytic approach, or what is culture for? In *Psychoanalytic Interpretations of Organizational Cultures*. Papers published by the International Society for the Psychoanalytic Study of Organizations.

Thompson, Michael G. (1990). College admissions: Failed rite of passage. Independent School Magazine. Winter.

Winnicott, D. W. (1965). *The Maturational Processes and the Facilitating Environment*. New York: International Universities Press.

T - #0601 - 101024 - C0 - 229/152/7 - PB - 9780789002235 - Gloss Lamination